The Healthy Lunchbox

How to Plan,
Prepare & Pack Stress-Free
Meals Kids Will Love

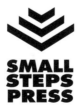

SMALL
STEPS
PRESS

Marie McClendon, MEd, and Cristy Shauck

Publisher, John Fedor; *Managing Editor, Book Publishing,* Abe Ogden; *Associate Director, Consumer Books,* Robert Anthony; *Manager, Book Production,* Melissa Sprott; *Illustration,* Lea Clark; *Composition,* Melissa Sprott; *Cover Design,* Pixiedesign; *Printer,* Worzalla Publishing.

Printed in the United States of America
1 3 5 7 9 10 8 6 4 2

Small Steps Press is an imprint of the American Diabetes Association. For information about Small Steps Press or the American Diabetes Association, in English or Spanish, call 1-800-342-2383. To order other Small Steps books, call 1-800-232-6733.

Consult a health care professional before trying any of the suggestions in this publication. Small Steps Press and ADA assume no responsibility for any injury that may result from the suggestions or information in this publication.

⊗ The paper in this publication meets the requirements of the ANSI Standard Z39.48-1992 (permanence of paper).

Small Steps Press titles may be purchased for business or promotional use or for special sales. To purchase this book in large quantities, or for custom editions of this book with your logo, contact Lee Romano Sequeira, Special Sales & Promotions, at the address below, or at Lees@smallstepspress.com or 703-299-2046.

Small Steps Press
1701 North Beauregard Street
Alexandria, Virginia 22311

Library of Congress Cataloging-in-Publication Data

McClendon, Marie.
The healthy lunchbox : quick, stress-free lunches kids will love / Marie McClendon, with Cristy Shauck.
p. cm.
Includes bibliographical references and index.
ISBN 1-58040-240-2 (alk. paper)
1. Lunchbox cookery. I. Shauck, Cristy. II. Title.

TX735.M43 2005
641.5'34--dc22

2005025307

For my sister, Linda.
Her body had diabetes and her spirit loved children.
—Marie

To Bill, Seth, and Elisabeth.
—Cristy

Table of Contents

Preface

Inspiration for writing this book came from a desperate attempt to get away from the dull and often unsatisfying pattern of packing tuna or peanut-butter-and-jelly sandwiches for four children. The quest for less stress on school mornings led to a library search of lunchbox guidebooks, but there weren't many choices that included mainly whole foods and excluded high-calorie, high-fat sweets. The goal was to change the frustration of hit-and-miss lunch-packing style into an organized, streamlined, and more enjoyable daily routine for the entire family. Other parents said they would love to get their hands on such a book, so after five years of learning to (somewhat) overcome too little time, lots of interruptions, and no small bit of self-doubt, this book was born.

Written by parents and edited by dietitians with experience packing nutrition-ally sound lunches that kids will actually eat, our mission included pumping some fun into the process. We've also included a variety of meals for kids with special eating needs, such as those with diabetes, food allergies, celiac disease, or just a few extra pounds.

Recipes have been tested on children and parents—both gave them two thumbs up. Sprinkled throughout are jokes, cartoons, graphics, quips, and quotes—that spoonful of sugar, if you will, to help the message go down.

Acknowledgements

With a full heart, we thank everyone who joined in this project to improve the health of future generations in a fun way. May all those mentioned below and all the unsung heroes know we appreciate all they did.

For their recipe contributions we'd like to thank newly retired teacher Sandy Kinro; Lauri Randolph, who has published two cookbooks; Russ Pencin, a fantastic cook; Jean C. Wade, a diabetic cookbook author; and Carol Fenster, Ph.D., an advocate for gluten-free diets. We're grateful to Leslie Noyes for editing support. Thanks to the librarians in Denver and Golden, Colorado, and numerous nutritionists. Many thanks to editor, Abe Ogden, for his humor, direction, words of support, and balancing of the female energy! A standing ovation to Lea Clark, our very talented young artist, for providing illustrations beyond her years.

Thanks to all the employees and customers at Mission Trace Vitamin Cottage who shared what their kids like best. A dozen roses to certified nutritionists Karen Falbo and Kelly Magill for their valuable expertise.

A special thank you from Cristy goes to her husband, Bill, for his loving support and expert computer and editing skills. Thanks also goes to her mom, Barbara Cowan, for testing recipes and keeping a loving eye on Cristy's daughter so Cristy could work on the manuscript. Thank you, Elisabeth, dear, for many hugs and kisses.

Thanks to Marie's 12-year-old sons, Jacob and Paul, for baking and fine-tuning countless recipes. Thanks to Jeff, Jacob, Paul, Anna, and Scott for taste testing when not always in the mood; for transforming dirty laundry to clean; for serving daddy duty; for computer wizardry; for doing extra chores; for much needed breaks playing cards; for great artwork and illustrations; and for patience, love, and faith.

Throughout this project there was the influence of Marie's sister. For help from the other side, thank you, Linda.

Introduction

"The message I really would like out there is that yes, a low-fat diet is good. But I would like to see people equally act on the recommendation for whole grains and fresh fruits and vegetables. A lot of people are eating low-fat prepared foods that are largely white flour and sugars. There are quick ways to make fresh produce tasty and eye-catching."
— Diane Moyer, MS, RD, CDE

"Emphasize to readers that diet is a matter of developing a healthy sense and instinct for what the body needs and to follow that, not a diet."
— Dr. Philip Incao, MD
Denver Family Physician

It's a little bit of an understatement to say that everyone is busy these days, especially families. Between school, work, soccer practices, chores, and a horde of other small responsibilities, it seems like there's never enough time. Unfortunately, as a society, it's our collective waistline that's paying the price. We turn to faster, unhealthier foods. We often don't take the time to exercise and most of us more often reach for the remote control instead of controlling our get-up-and-go. And we're passing this legacy on to our children. Obesity among youngsters is skyrocketing, children are being diagnosed with type 2 diabetes (once considered an adult disease), and for the first time in as long as anyone can remember, researchers are saying that the average lifespan for the current generation of Americans will actually be shorter than the generation before. Yikes.

It's a little sobering, isn't it? Well, not to worry. We're not here to scare the pants off of you. Things aren't as bad as all that. There's a very popular myth out there that eating good food is complicated or time consuming, that fixing healthy meals for a family is a constant chore, especially those slapdash meals we stuff into lunchboxes or cooler bags every morning. That myth is plain wrong. Not only can good-for-you lunches be put together quickly and easily, they can do even more. We designed this book with the idea that you can transform lunch-packing into a cooperative, family effort that reaps several rewards: less stress, family bonding opportunities, healthier lunches, and thus healthier kids who learn lifetime good eating habits.

The important thing is to get the whole family involved. Not only does this make your job easier, but we've also found that when children have some say or put effort into making their own take-along lunch, they are more likely to eat it. And, as our studies have shown, actually eating the food helps kids get the nutrients packed inside!

Possible Outcomes from Reading Our Amazing Book

- More food into your child and less into the trashcan
- The magical appearance of nutritionally sound, tasty meals from recipes and menus for school lunches, including some gluten-free, dairy-free, and vegetarian main dishes
- Effective methods to help your kids combat junk food jealousy
- A heckuva' lot less stress on school mornings

What You'll Find in This Book

- A handy rotation menu for no-brainer planning in the morning
- Tips for interviewing your children about their food likes and dislikes and follow-up
- Effective ways to combat junk food jealousy in a non-confrontational way
- Tips for training your children to pack their own nutritious lunch
- Hints for stocking and organizing your pantry and refrigerator to make them kid-friendly
- Tips for money-saving lunches and convenient pre-packaged foods
- A few unusual ideas
- Resources, children's books, and product sources

Disclaimer

We assembled this book with the goal of honoring as many lifestyles as possible. A few of our ideas may be too "granola" or "brown rice" for some people, and a few ideas may be too "fast food" for others. If so, try not to let a few ideas keep you from taking advantage of the rest. Think of it as a smorgasbord—take what you like and skip what you don't.

Some Helpful Tools

Like any effort worth undertaking, proper planning and a good set of tools pave the way for tasty packed lunches. We recommend a few items that will speed up the food preparation process:

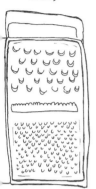

- Apple slicer
- Food processor (a good one lasts a very long time)
  - Coffee grinder reserved just for seeds and grains (be sure to brush and shake it out between uses)
  - Good mixer
  - Child-friendly grater

When you have the time, use kitchen tools powered by elbow grease and not electricity. Going manual not only means the kids can help, but it's also a little extra exercise automatically slipped into the day—exercise that produces something tasty.

Notes on the Recipes

To find recipes that are quick to prepare, or those without gluten or dairy, look for special icons (see page 56 for icon guide). Using the indexes at the beginning of each section is also quick way to find what you want.

In some of the recipes, we list different options for different ingredients. The first ingredient listed was usually our choice for either nutritional reasons or taste preference. But it's always nice to have choices. Be sensitive to your own family's tastes and consider what's in the pantry, too.

One Last Thing
Before We Get Started...

The ideas presented herein are not a guarantee of family bliss and health. But if they work, praise our book to the Heavens and buy copies for your friends, relatives, and schools!

Illustrations courtesy Paul McClendon, Age 12.

Part One: Get Ready!

Chapter One: Do You Like Green Beans and Spam?
Discovering Your Child's Favorite Foods and Strong Dislikes

Chapter Two: Nutrition Nitty Gritty
A Crash Course in Nutrition Basics

Chapter Three: Applying What You've Learned
Tips and Tricks for Turning Nutrition Knowledge into Healthy Reality

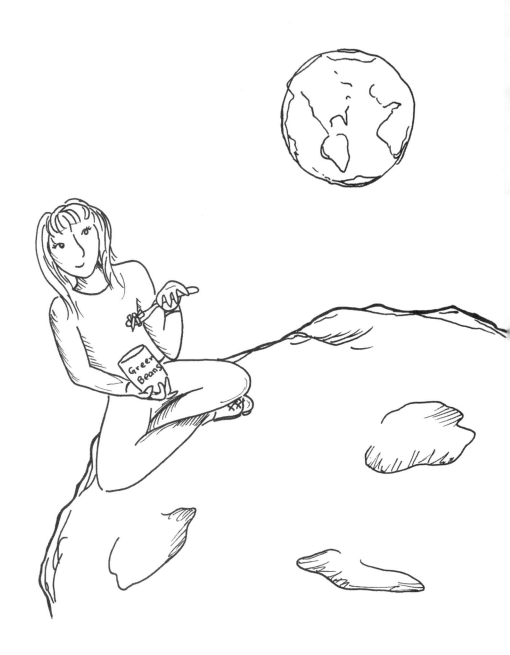

Chapter One
Do You Like Green Beans and Spam?

Discovering Your Child's Favorite Foods and Strong Dislikes

> Do you like green beans and spam?
> Would you eat them steamed?
> Would you eat them creamed?
> Would you eat them with a spoon?
> Would you eat them on the moon?
> Would you eat them with a pear?
> Would you eat them *anywhere*?

This book is dedicated to helping parents get good food into their children without a lot of headache. With that in mind, we've tried to fill these pages with tips and tricks that make packing healthy lunches a snap. But no amount of clever packaging will promote healthy eating if what you're packing *never gets eaten*. So before we get into whipping up recipes or explaining nutrition therapy (trust us, it's not as dry as it sounds), we should address the most important aspect of our entire approach: What do your kids like to eat?

An Interview?

Giving kids what they like is the easiest way to make sure they will actually eat it. But what does your child like that you can say yes to? We parents like to think we know everything about our kids, but often you can be surprised by what you don't know. It may sound a little formal, but an interview can be a great way to find out what kids crave. It can be as casual as asking kids to point out foods they like while strolling down the grocery aisles, as elaborate as setting up a formal interview with a questionnaire, or as covert as watching what they order and enjoy in restaurants. No matter how you approach it, there are some important factors to keep in mind.

- Timing is the key to success. Take advantage of lulls in activity times or when you'd be talking with your children anyway. Pulling your child away from the swing set to talk about lunches probably won't work too well.

- Choose the location carefully. Avoid distractions, or take advantage of outside cues to work the conversation in naturally (such as at the supermarket or in a restaurant).

- Ask for the top favorites in each food group. A shortcut is to ask what they would trade for at school.

- Sometimes you may not be the best person for the job. Depending on the mood, the best interviewer might be Mom, Dad, Grandma, a neighbor, or even another child.

News to Me

"I really like that warm homemade almond milk we have for breakfast."

– Marie's daughter Anna, during an interview

"Sure surprised me."

– Marie's reaction

You know your kids best, so the way you set up the interview is up to you. Following are some of the methods we've found actually work.

The supermarket stroll

Conducting the interview at a grocery store is a great approach for kids who need to see, smell, and touch the real thing. Actually having something tangible in front of them can be a great way to get them interacting and volunteering information. Some things to keep in mind:

- If you try this during a normal shopping trip, allow extra time for discussion and examination of foods.

- This method is especially good for kids who shrug their shoulders and aren't big talkers.

- Take it a little at a time. One or two departments per trip may be plenty for most kids.

- If you have more than one youngster to feed, focus on one child at a time if possible (twins and other multiples may do better together).
- Avoid the meat department. Ground beef and raw chicken drumsticks don't look very appetizing. Cruise down the frozen food aisle or by the deli department to give your kids an idea of how meat will appear in the lunchbox.

Where do you steer your shopping cart?

Have you noticed the healthiest foods run along the outside aisles of the supermarket? The produce, the dairy, the meat, the eggs.... Now think about the inside aisles and the boxed products lining the shelves. Next time you're grabbing groceries, "drive" your shopping cart through healthier neighborhoods.

Car trips

During those long stretches down the interstate, an interview can be a great way to pass the time. The end of summer vacation before school lunches start up again may be ideal, but any time is fine. Naturally, the interviewer should be a non-driver who takes notes or tape-records the child's responses. On a road trip to a family reunion, Marie's family recorded their first interview in a small notebook. They still have fun reviewing and adding new favorites.

Save it for a rainy day

Or a snow day, or a vacation day, or anytime the kids are in the house anyway. Avoid making it seem like a chore by setting a relaxed mood using some of the suggestions below.

- Read a related children's book together, like *Green Eggs and Ham* or *D.W. the Picky Eater*.
- Let older kids choose and make a rainy day snack (which in itself reveals at least one food preference) before beginning the interview.
- Get cozy on the couch or chat over hot cocoa and cookies.

Helpful suggestions:

- Let the child know the discussion can stop at any time. Watch for signs that the child is losing interest. It's better to stop before hearing, "Are we done yet?" or "I don't want to do this anymore." And if you don't have perfect radar that day, perhaps shrug your shoulders and continue another day.
- If the situation gets a little confrontational, ask relatives, friends, or neighbors what your child eats at their homes. Or ask an adult to call, e-mail, or instant message the child for the interview.

Do You Like Green Beans and Spam? 9

- One way to get the conversation ball rolling is to share some childhood favorites or dislikes of your own before asking kids to share theirs. Or say enthusiastically, "Guess what I had for lunch?"
- Add splashes of laughter.
- Interview with a makeshift or a real microphone and tape recorder to keep the child's attention and record the findings. If you're feeling especially enthusiastic, you can dress up for the part. Playing a waiter or a waitress could be easy and fun, too.
- Ask what they like to receive in a lunch trade. What have they seen other kids bring for lunch that they'd like to try? Naturally, we're trying to cut down on trading by giving them something they wouldn't want to part with, but lunchroom bartering is still always fun.
- Simply try new dishes for dinner before packing them away in lunch boxes. Just watching what and how much they eat gives accurate feedback without overdoing the opinion game.

Handy Charts for the Interviewing Process

Following are some helpful charts you can use during your interviews to record your child's preferences. Fill in blank rows with favorites not listed. We placed common food items in five groups:

- Fruits
- Vegetables (we know, tomatoes are a fruit, but we put them in here because they're more often used as vegetables)
- Dairy Products and Non-Dairy Substitutes
- Protein: Meats, Poultry, Fish, Eggs, and Other Sources
- Main Dishes, Salads, and Snacks

Fruits

Food name	Like	Don't like	Will try
apples (write in the specific varieties)			
apricots			
avocados			
bananas			
blackberries			
blueberries			
cantaloupe			
cherries			
coconut			
dates			
figs			
grapefruit			
grapes			
honeydew melon			
kiwi fruit			
lemon			
lime			
mango			
nectarines			
oranges			
papayas			
peaches			
pears			
persimmon			
pineapple			
plantains			
plums			
pomegranate			
raisins			
star fruit			
strawberries			
tangelo			
tangerines			
watermelon			

Vegetables

Food name	Like	Don't like	Will try
artichoke			
asparagus			
bean sprouts			
beets			
Bell peppers: red, yellow, green			
broccoli			
Brussels sprouts			
cabbage			
carrots			
cauliflower			
celery			
collards			
corn			
cucumbers			
eggplant			
green beans			
jicama			
kale			
kohlrabi			
leeks			
lettuce			
onions			
parsnips			
potatoes			
pumpkin			
snap peas			
soybeans			
spinach			
squash			
sweet potatoes, yams			
tomatoes			
turnips			
watercress			

Dairy Products and Non-Dairy Substitutes

Food name	Like	Don't like	Will try
butter			
cheeses (almost endless varieties)			
cottage cheeses			
cream cheeses			
milk			
sour cream			
soy (milk, yogurt, cheeses, etc.)			
yogurt			

Protein: Meats, Poultry, Fish, Eggs, and Other Sources

Food name	Like	Don't like	Will try
Beef			
hamburger			
steak			
stew beef			
short ribs			
roast beef			
Chicken/Turkey			
thigh			
breast			
wing			
drumstick			
nuggets			
tenders			
canned chunks			
Eggs			
scrambled			
fried			
soft boiled			
hard boiled			
omelets			
poached			
Fish			
sticks			
fillets			
canned tuna/salmon			
Nuts			
peanuts			
cashews			
pecans			
pistachios			
pine nuts			
almonds			
chestnuts			
hazelnuts			
nut butters			

Food name	Like	Don't like	Will try
Pork			
chops			
bacon			
ribs			
sausage			
ham			
Seeds			
sunflower seeds			
pumpkin seeds			
poppy seeds			
sesame seeds			
Other			
tofu			
tempeh			
soynuts			

Main Dishes, Salads, and Snacks

Food name	Like	Don't like	Will try
casseroles			
chili			
fruit salad			
pasta salad			
sandwiches			
soup			
veggie salad			
wraps			

Chapter Two
Nutrition Nitty Gritty
A Crash Course in Nutrition Basics

With a little planning, lunchbox lunches can be well-balanced, tasty, and appealing. We promise. And most of the time, it doesn't require reinventing the wheel. Many recipes in this book have been adapted to lower the fat, sugar, and salt content of some old favorites (but we also had a blast inventing some new family winners).

Maybe you've already had a chance to sit down with your child and talk about their likes and dislikes (in which case, we commend you on jumping right in). Maybe not. Doing this is a big first step, but it is just the first. Now you need to get up to speed on what actually makes a healthy lunch and how you can start crafting some of your own. If your kids say they love Twinkies and hot dogs (and no surprises if they do), it's going to take a little work to bridge the gap between the sweet, fatty concoctions they crave and foods that are good for their bodies as well as their taste buds.

We'll start with some nutrition basics. Consider this information the foundation to your healthy lunchbox creations.

Nutrition 101—The Basics

Right out of the gate, a little heads up—nutrition science is constantly progressing, evolving, and changing (part of the reason so many throw up their hands in frustration). For decades, fats were seen as the bad guys. Not necessarily true. While we know that *trans* fats are bad guys, we also know that monounsaturated fats and omega-3 fatty acids are essential cornerstones of a healthy diet.

More recently, carbohydrates have come under fire and we've seen an explosion in fad diets that tout high-protein, low-carb meal plans. While processed sugars and other nutrient-deprived carbs are in fact leading to a lot of extra calories in the American belly, good carbs, such as those in vegetables and whole grains, are absolutely necessary. There is always going to be new "breakthrough" research that contradicts the previous "breakthrough" research into how the body processes certain foods, as well as new recommendations on what it is we should be eating. However, even as the details and fine particulars shift around, there are some principles about foods that stay the same.

Three types of nutrients come loaded with the energy, or calories, our bodies process to move, think, breathe, and generally stay alive—carbohydrates, fats, and proteins. These three groups keep us going. Everyone also needs a variety of vitamins and minerals to provide support for the energy-packed big three.

Carbohydrates feed your brain!

You've probably been hearing a lot about carbohydrates these days, and more often than not, what you read or hear from one source contradicts what you read or hear from another. For some experts, carbs are the source of all dietary evil; for others, they're the nutritious foundation for a healthy meal plan. To some degree, both camps are right. Because of all the confusion, we're going to give carbohydrates a little more attention.

There are three main types of carbohydrate—starch, sugar, and fiber. To get an idea of how carbs can be both good and bad, we'll look at each form a little more closely.

Starch

All-natural starches are often the healthiest form of carbohydrate, and include such foods as peas, potatoes, dried beans, lentils, and grains. While a pea is a pea and a bean is a bean, grains can be a little trickier. Take wheat, for example. Wheat contains three parts—the bran, germ, and the endosperm. When all of these parts are together you consider this whole-grain wheat. If you eat a whole-grain food, you get all of the nutrients that whole grains have to offer. If you eat a refined-grain food, it contains only the endosperm, or the starchy part, so you miss out on a lot of vitamins and minerals. Reading the ingredient list is the easiest way to tell if a food is made from whole grains. Look for the first ingredient to be whole-wheat flour, brown rice, rye flour, barley, or oats. You'll also want to avoid enriched wheat flour as much as possible. Enriched wheat flour is a refined grain—sometimes listed as all-purpose flour, cake flour, bleached flour, and bread flour—and is not nearly as healthy as whole grains. You find it in most brand-name breads, as well as in baked products such as cake, cookies, muffins, and snack bars. Often, products that used enriched wheat flour have added sugar and fat. These are called processed foods. A good rule of thumb, especially for grains, is that the further away a food is from its natural state, the less nutritious it is.

Sugar

Sugar is another type of carbohydrate and there are two main types: naturally occurring sugars, such as those in milk or fruit, and added sugars, such as those added during processing of snack cakes, colas, and heavy-syrup canned fruit. It doesn't take a nutrition genius to figure out which of these two types you'll want to avoid. Foods with added sugar are usually higher in calories and fat and lower in other nutrients, such as fiber, vitamins, and minerals. Also, as surprising as this may sound, a lot of foods that tout themselves as "healthy" are pumped full of added sugars. Many low-fat foods use sugar to replace the taste lost when they drop the fat content. Because of this, a low-fat diet can actually sabotage weight loss when a person eats more carbs to feel full. Obviously, eating foods with added sugar is perfectly acceptable as long as it's done in moderation. Paying attention to what

A little about the
Glycemic Index

You may have heard something about the glycemic index. Or maybe not. Basically, this is just a ranking of carbohydrate-containing foods, based on how quickly this food will raise glucose (sugar) levels in the blood. This has a little more meaning for kids and adults with diabetes, who need to match their medicine with their blood glucose levels, but it also is important for others because it indicates how your body metabolizes certain foods. Some research has indicated that foods with a higher glycemic index (that raise blood glucose quicker) may be unhealthier. Unfortunately, the index can be confusing at best. Some foods that seem like they would have a low index, like rice, actually have a very high index. And when you combine certain foods together, it can change their index rankings completely. As a whole, studying the glycemic index and trying to cut down on foods that raise blood glucose quickly wouldn't hurt. But until more research is done, this isn't the meal planning tool it may become in the future.

you and your family are eating is the key to avoiding a lot of extra sugar. Check ingredients for things like sugar, turbinado, maple syrup, high-fructose corn syrup, and sugar cane syrup. You'll be surprised how many foods have been pumped with sugar. Almost every sliced bread on the market, for example, is juiced up with high-fructose corn syrup. You may also see sugars listed by their chemical names. You can recognize these sugars on labels because their chemical names end in "-ose," for example glucose (also called dextrose), fructose (also called levulose), lactose, and maltose. Sometimes, food companies get sneaky and list a variety of different sugars to avoid having to list sugar at the beginning of the list (where the most-used ingredients have to go). Keep an eye out for this, as well.

A Sweet Alternative—Agave Nectar

This may take a little bit of tracking down, but a great alternative sweetener available in health food stores is agave nectar, which comes from the agave plant. It looks and tastes something like honey, only less sweet and less thick. It pours easily and goes farther on pancakes than maple syrup. It's a fine substitute for honey in baking, too.

Research: For an interesting tour of sugars found around the world, go to *www.foodsubs.com/Sweeten.html.* Keep in mind that we don't endorse any of the alternatives nor can we support any claims about any suggested health benefits of the sugars discussed. But it's always nice to know what's out there. For other options Marie's family enjoys, go to *www.wholehumanbeans.com.*

Fiber

Fiber is the part of plant foods—fruits, vegetables, whole grains, nuts, and beans—we can't digest. Unfortunately, we as a country don't eat nearly enough fiber. When you eat dietary fiber, most of it passes through the intestines undigested. Why is this important? Because not only does it help promote regularity (you know what we're talking about), it also helps your kids feel full and satisfied without adding calories and leaving them wanting more food. Good sources of dietary fiber include:

• fruits and vegetables
• whole grains
• beans and legumes
• nuts

In general, it's best to get fiber from food rather than taking a supplement (though we doubt you'll be dropping fiber supplements into lunchboxes anytime soon). Not only do you get the fiber from high-fiber foods, but these nutritious selections are usually packed with many important vitamins and minerals. In fact, they may contain healthy nutrients that haven't even been discovered yet!

USA Stands for Unrelentingly Sweetened America

Can you guess the average sugar intake for the average American? 32 teaspoons per day—about 2/3 of a cup!

That's 650 calories a day and almost 250,000 calories in a year. A quarter of a million calories in a year! Keep track of your sugar sipping and supping per day and set goalposts. Aim for about 10 teaspoons a day at the most. And be careful of too much sugar in beverages. Kids can drink a lot of calories without even knowing it. Sugar is sneaky.

Keep in mind that you'll want to increase fiber intake gradually. Stuffing a lunch with lots of fiber right away will leave your kids doubled over with stomach irritation and constipation. That can make for a very uncomfortable recess.

Fats aren't always the bad guys

Not too long ago, fats were fingered in the nutrient lineup as the culprit of America's ballooning waistlines. We were told that if we cut out the fat, well, we won't be fat. Turns out, that's not necessarily the case. In fact, this advice may be part of the reason we're as plump as we are. Thinking that if we just avoided fats we could eat anything we want, Americans started scarfing down nonfat foods, such as fat-free frozen yogurt and baked potato chips. Guess what? These foods still have calories, and because there's no fat to make you feel full, you can eat a heck of a lot more of them. Fat or no, a bag of potato chips is still swimming with calories, and it doesn't matter where they come from—all unburned calories are stored as fat in the body.

So, we're telling you point blank—eat fats. Make a third of the calories your family eats fat. But—and this is a huge but—eat good ones and keep an eye on calories. Cut down on saturated fats because these fats are filled with cholesterol. Run kicking and screaming as far away as you can from *trans* fats. These are highly processed fats that raise LDL (bad) cholesterol levels and lower HDL (good) levels. If you see *trans* fat on the Nutrition Facts label (a new, shopper-friendly requirement) or "partially-hydrogenated oil" in the ingredient list of a package, set it down and slowly back away. A good rule of thumb? If the food is in a box and has fat, it's almost always going to be the wrong kind.

So which fats have the right stuff? Monounsaturated and polyunsaturated fats, the kind you find in healthy oils and fish, are the fats of choice. These guys raise your HDL cholesterol levels (that's good cholesterol) and add flavor and a filling quality to food. Plus, they're good for the skin and hair (always a plus for those appearance-conscious adolescent years). Rich sources of good fats include:

- avocados
- peanut butter
- fish—packed with super healthy omega-3 fatty acids, but see the box *Finding (surprising chemicals in) Nemo*

Finding (surprising chemicals in) Nemo

Fish is good food. It's packed with omega-3 fatty acids and is an excellent source of protein. Unfortunately, especially in bottom feeders and fish that feed on other fish, it can also be packed with unhealthy levels of mercury. If you're thinking about packing fish into lunches, limit it to about once a week. Otherwise, you might be packing more than you'd like.

- nuts
- vegetable oils, such as olive oil and canola oil
- even mayonnaise (but watch the calories!)

Proteins—the building blocks of the body

Put simply, proteins are the raw materials out of which our bodies our built. They work together to form bone, muscle, cartilage, skin, and blood, as well as important enzymes, hormones, and vitamins. Without proteins, our bodies simply would not work. Foods heavy in protein include meats, legumes, and dairy. However, you can get protein from sources other than animals.

If you or your child prefers to not eat meat or dairy, rest assured that you can still get plenty of proteins, though it takes a little more planning and thought. It was once assumed that combining certain legumes and grains in different ways in the same meal helped mimic essential amino acids (the building blocks of proteins), and thus was a better way of gobbling up vegetarian protein. We now know that this is not true—protein is protein. Focus on eating a variety of different non-animal proteins throughout the day. If you or your children are lacto-ovo vegetarians and don't mind eating dairy and eggs, these are excellent sources of protein. Other sources of non-animal proteins include

- beans
- nuts
- nut butters, such as peanut butter
- peas
- soy products, such as tofu and tempeh

Vitamins and minerals—the supporting cast

Vitamins and minerals aren't nutrients like protein, carbohydrate, and fat, because they don't contain any calories. However, these guys are essential for a healthy, well-functioning body, especially in growing children. Think of them as the extra actors in the ongoing show of a functioning body. Nutrients like carbs and fats have snatched the lead roles, but vitamins and minerals are what make the whole production work. Each vitamin and mineral plays a different role and all are essential. You can get a lot of these vitamins and minerals in supplements and pills, but it's generally better to get your vitamins in their natural state; that is, in food. Luckily, good foods, such as leafy greens and dairy foods, usually bundle them up for easy eating.

Vitamin B

Our bodies need more than twelve different B vitamins alone. Some are in grains, some are in meat, and some are in green leafy vegetables. They are good for muscles, nerves, skin, the blood system, even the tongue.

Vitamin C

Vitamin C is good for teeth, bones, the blood system, muscles, gums, and skin. It's in citrus fruits, melons, Brussels sprouts, cabbage, berries, green leafy vegetables, turnips, lima beans, potatoes, asparagus, winter squash, green peas, and cauliflower.

Vitamin A

Vitamin A is good for eyes, bones, skin, and teeth, as well as the mucous linings of the body. Greens like spinach, cooked tomatoes, dried apricots, peaches, pumpkin, carrots, and eggs contain this vitamin. In the United States, Vitamin A is also added to the milk we buy.

Vitamin D

Vitamin D is good for bones, so it's important for growing bodies. It's in eggs, liver, and some fish. Like vitamin A, it's also added to milk.

Vitamin E

Vitamin E helps keep every cell healthy. It's mainly in vegetable oils, nuts, seeds, and wheat germ.

Vitamin K

Vitamin K helps blood clot and form a scab when we get a cut. Sources of it are green leafy vegetables, the cabbage family, liver, and soybeans.

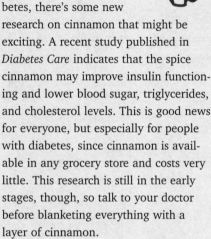

We Propose a Cinnamon Toast

Really bad jokes aside, if you've got a child with diabetes, there's some new research on cinnamon that might be exciting. A recent study published in *Diabetes Care* indicates that the spice cinnamon may improve insulin functioning and lower blood sugar, triglycerides, and cholesterol levels. This is good news for everyone, but especially for people with diabetes, since cinnamon is available in any grocery store and costs very little. This research is still in the early stages, though, so talk to your doctor before blanketing everything with a layer of cinnamon.

Most Americans consider cinnamon a sweet spice and include it in baked goods like cookies, pies, and cakes. But other cultures use it in meat and poultry dishes. In the Mediterranean, it's in moussaka, a tomato-based eggplant-and-meat casserole with an egg-and-cheese sauce. In Arabic countries, it's in chicken biryani, a sort of chicken pie. It's also found in the Mexican spicy ground beef dish called picadillo. Cristy's family sprinkles it on French toast, yams, sweet potatoes, and oatmeal, too.

Minerals

We also need a variety of minerals, which are also readily available in good, healthy foods. To name just a few: calcium (for bones and teeth, muscles, nerves, and blood); potassium; sodium; magnesium iron; zinc; and selenium.

Some Tricks of the Nutrition Trade

If you want to get the most nutrition out of food, think fresh and whole.
Does the food you're about to eat look like it does in nature? If so, you're on
the right track. The water content in whole foods is filling. For the most
part, fruits and vegetables (washed and rinsed, of course) may be eaten
raw. When some vegetables are boiled, vitamins can partially leach out into
the cooking water, so steaming is preferable. But if you do boil, you can
always save the water for soup.

We can't stress whole grains enough. Whole-grain breakfast cereals and
breads offer fiber and more vitamins and minerals than their paler, refined
equivalents. Same goes for rolled oats, which are healthier than minute
oats. Regular Cream of Wheat has more fiber than the quick version. Read
labels and compare.

We are made of about 98% water.
We need to drink lots of it daily. Guess what? If we don't drink enough
water, our bodies begin getting dehydrated and we stop working properly.
Adults need to drink 8-10 glasses of water daily—more in some climates or
if you've done a lot of exercise. Kids may not need this much. Talk with
your family doctor to see how much your kids should be drinking. If adding
a little flavor helps, try putting in a bit of lemon or lime.

Drinking soda pop doesn't count as drinking water.
For a couple of reasons. First, soda has caffeine, which is a diuretic that
causes your body to become dehydrated. In other words, you don't get any
of the hydrating effects of water. Second, soda is either chock full of sugar
(and thus, calories kids don't need) or artificial sweeteners. Most kids drink
waayyyy too many calories as a whole, so anything you can do to cut down
on these "invisible" calories is a step in the right direction.

Chapter Three
Applying What You've Learned

Tips and Tricks for Turning Nutrition
Knowledge into Healthy Reality

Before we move on to the daunting architecture, psychology, and diplomacy that can be packing lunches for your kids, it's time for some applied nutrition. We want healthy foods in our kids' bellies, right? Here are a few tricks and tips to help make sure all of the stuff we talked about in the last chapter gets to its intended destination.

Nature's Candy?
Believe Us, They're Not Buying it

Most kids aren't getting enough fruits and vegetables, and they sure as heck don't go out of their way to start. So it's up to you to make sure their diets are nutrient rich. Following are a few tips to make this a little easier.

- The recommended amount of servings of vegetables a day is five. Which seems like a huge amount, but is definitely still doable. A serving of vegetables is 1/2 cup veggies or 3/4 cup vegetable juice. The amount of vegetables in a main dish or even muffin (think zucchini, corn, carrots) also counts. If you want to get creative (or downright sneaky), chop cooked broccoli fine as a frog's eyelash and slip it into spaghetti sauce or lasagna.

- Use color as a quick visual guide for deciding whether the meal is balanced, or at least colorful. Is there something green? Something orange? Red? Yellow?
- Think combinations. Children will often eat veggies with a dipping sauce, which can be as simple as diluted ranch dressing on the side. They may hate carrots, but love carrot-raisin salad.
- When it comes to fruit, especially for younger kids, think bite-size and fun dips.
- Combine apples with carrots in grated salad; add cabbage for a fruity coleslaw.
- Never underestimate the power of campy Australians in colorful shirts. Our hats are off to that zany group, the Wiggles, for their lively rendition of "Fruit Salad, Yummy, Yummy." This inspired kids across the world to ask for this delicious way to get plenty of vitamins and minerals.

Table 3-1. Healthy Substitutes for Unhealthy Favorites

Unhealthy Favorite	Healthy Substitute
Breaded chicken nuggets	Cooked chicken cubes with low-fat dipping sauce
Chips	Baked chips, rice cakes, corn thins
Doughnuts	Homemade low-fat muffins and cookies
French fries	Oven fries, veggies and dipping sauce
Fruit leather (roll-ups)	100% fruit leather
Regular hot dogs, bologna	Low-fat versions without nitrates, additives, or food coloring
Soda and juice-flavored drinks	milk, water, 100% juice, occasional Kool Aid with 1/2 cup granulated fructose
Pre-packaged lunches	English muffin pizza, cheese and crackers in fun containers
Toaster pastries	Muffin with 100% fruit preservatives
Cookies, cakes, pastries	Low-fat versions with healthier sweeteners
Crackers	Non-trans-fat, whole-grain crackers
Milk shake	Smoothies
Nachos	Melted cheese between two tortillas in wedges
Buttered popcorn	Lightly buttered or seasoned popcorn
Potato salad	Sweet potato salad
Salad dressing	Homemade Thousand Island dressing (mayonnaise and salsa)
Jell-O®	Fruit juice plus unflavored gelatin and fruit

Exercise: An Underused Therapy

If you saw an ad for a pill that made you feel better, helped you lose weight even though you ate more, helped you build muscle, evened your mood, eliminated insomnia, and sub-stantially helped prevent the number one killer of Americans today (heart disease), you'd buy 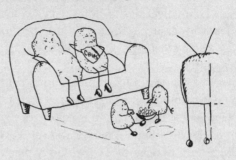 them by the bucketful, wouldn't you? You see where this is going. Exercise is the best medicine for humans on the market today. Perhaps someday doctors will write out prescriptions for exercise and coordinate with organizations, such as health clubs, sports programs, swimming pools, and dance studios, to hand out "samples" of day passes like they do with prescription drugs. Perhaps someday health insurance could cover prescribed exercise for those who need to lose weight. Makes financial sense, doesn't it? Cover a few bucks now on exercise to save thousands on claims for hospital and doctor bills down the road. Unfortunately, the health care industry hasn't caught on yet. Until then, remember that exercise is the number one best thing you can do as a family. Your body simply works better when it's in shape, whether you're six years old or sixty. Healthy eating can only go so far. Just look at the new USDA guidelines—half of the recommendations are for exercise! We understand that getting enough activity can be tough, but this is also when families can have the most fun. Turn off the TV, lay down the video game controllers, step away from the computer, and get outside and be active. Play soccer, throw around a baseball, ride bikes, take the dog for a long walk, just do something. Not only will you be setting a great precedent for your children, but you'll be helping yourself as well.

Fun Indoor/Outdoor Exercises

- Safe, respectful roughhousing with supervision: tickle, wrestle, tag
- Exercise class with a best friend
- Mini trampoline (to music)
- Hula hoop
- Jump rope

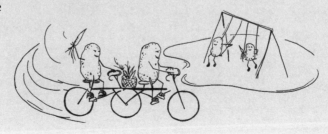

A Few Healthy Preparation Ideas

- Use whole-wheat pastry flour, which you can find in health food stores, whenever possible. We tried it in our recipe for muffins (in Section 3) and they rose just as high as with all-purpose.
- Use sprinkles whenever possible. They don't add much sugar and you'll be surprised how far a little presentation can go. Sprinkle over muffins and cookies before baking, so they stay on the food. Do this over a plate or waxed paper so you can re-use sprinkles.
- For a slightly different taste, substitute low-fat buttermilk for the milk in baking recipes. It goes well with any recipe that calls for apples or rhubarb.
- If you've got gluten concerns, try Pamela's Ultimate Baking & Pancake Mix. The leavening in this gluten-free product is equal to approximately 1 teaspoon baking powder and 1/4 teaspoon baking soda per cup.
- Serve quality veggies that are fresh. Kids seem to prefer crunch and the louder the better. Sometimes raw vegetables don't taste as bitter to a child's taste buds.

Part Two: Get Set!

Chapter Four: Pack that Delicious, Nutritious Lunch with Zen Tranquility
Your Guide to the Psychology, Diplomacy, and Architecture of the Lunchbox

Chapter Five: Mom, I Can't Find the Tuna!
Creating a Kid-Friendly Kitchen

Chapter Six: What about Breakfast?
*Grab-and-Go Grub for Breaking the Fast—
When They Have to Eat on the Run or Go Hungry*

Chapter Seven: This Isn't So Hard!
*Handy Menu Rotation Charts and a Lunchbox-Packing Blueprint
Guide to Keep the Lunch Packer on Track*

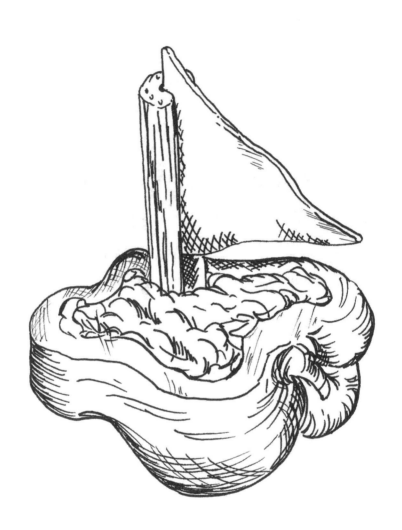

Chapter Four

Pack That Delicious, Nutritious Lunch with Zen Tranquility

Your Guide to the Psychology, Diplomacy, and Architecture of the Lunchbox

No other section in this book brought such agony and intimidation to your humble authors than the one you're reading now. Not only is this the real meat and bones of our lunchbox packing plan, it's also the wiliest part of the whole packed meal process. We all have a pretty good idea of what makes a healthy lunch (and if not, hopefully the last chapter shed a little light). But what good is that if the food sits stinking up a lunchbox? Here's where you need to break out the psychology. And this is tricky, unpredictable stuff. Sometimes it works; sometimes it bombs. Still, we boldly dared to tackle it.

In this chapter, we've included several suggestions for making food more appealing, but every family needs certain nutritional rules that kids must abide by. You can't be sneaky all the time and ground rules are an essential part of parenting. Think seatbelts. Kids don't like them, but once they realize the rule's not going to change and that there's a good reason behind it, they learn to accept it. As long as the rule's fair and consistent, kids eventually understand that it needs to be followed.

History Repeats Itself

*I so vividly remember my own childhood indignation—
40 years ago—about how my mother thought an
apple was dessert, and how I coveted the Hostess
Cupcakes that other people got. Until college, when I
had real freedom, and bought a package of cupcakes
and took one bite before realizing that it was really horrid,
and threw the rest away. I tried to give away the second cupcake (never one to waste "food"), but none of my fellow students would
take it! Now of course I get to re-live the entire experience. Except now I am
the evil mom.*   – Jean Rystrom
                          Pediatrics Specialty Service Manager for Kaiser Permanente

Junk Food Jealousy

Remember wanting a classmate's Hershey chocolate bar and having to catch
the drool on the way down? Guess what? Things haven't changed. Junk food
jealousy may be the biggest obstacle to healthy lunches, especially if eating
healthy is a new lunchtime trend. Staring across the table at another kid's
Snickers, chips, and soda may instigate some of these silent, and not so silent,
thoughts from your kids:

- "She gets more desserts than I do."
- "When did my parents decide they won't go within 10 feet of a Twinkie?"
- "Boy, that snack looks cool."
- "I feel left out."
- "Wonder if she'd notice if I took a little bite out of that."

Before listing numerous ways to make food more appealing, we want to say
that usually what the child misses is the *social experience of eating what peers
are eating* rather than the actual taste experience. Kids don't like to be left out
of the experiences of their peers (see the bazillion two-month fads you've
probably already gone through). On the flip side, kids *love* to be trendsetters.
If you can whip up meals that other kids drool over, just try and stop your
kids from eating them. It's your job, and it's a doozie, to help your kids first
understand that eating healthier is here to stay (think seatbelts), and second,
help bridge the gap so the jealousy bug doesn't bite quite as often.

Six ways to counter junk food jealousy

1. Get your child involved in the lunch-making process.

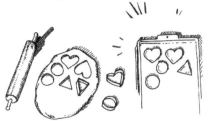

Kids are way more likely to eat food that they've prepared themselves. If they feel a sense of ownership, they have a tangible attachment to the healthier option.

2. Offer healthier substitutions that retain the spirit of the original.

Close counts in horseshoes, hand grenades, *and* packed lunches. See Table 3-1 on page 26 for a list of common favorites and a healthier version.

3. Find acceptable ways to trade.

Kids trade lunches just to trade. It's fun. It's a friendship thing. It's getting away from eating the same ol' things. Marie's daughter trades jerky for Jell-O. Must be a "J" thing! Ask your child what they like to trade and then you'll know what to pack for a high-quality food transaction. The thing to stress is "healthy food for healthy food." Let your kids know that if that homemade fruit leather is going for a candy bar, they got a bum deal. Nobody likes to be on the wrong end of a trade, or, shall we say, no *body* likes to be on the wrong end of a trade.

Kids who have special dietary concerns, like kids with diabetes or celiac disease, can trade, too. You just need to make sure the trades fit in nicely with their meal plans. Here are some tips for healthy free trade:

- Ask what foods get traded the most and pack them.
- Teach kids to make smart trades for their bodies. Trading a fruit for a fruit, an allowed snack for an allowed snack, or a protein for a protein.
- Tell your kids to keep the trading smooth or teachers and lunch monitors may outlaw the lunch stock exchange.
- Approach the parents of the children your children trade lunch with and brainstorm ways to make trading healthy for both families.

4. You can catch more kids with flavor than with fiber.

If you only buy whole grain macaroni and nobody eats it, you've won the battle and lost the war. Instead, buy what they want and sprinkle in fiber, such as oat bran, rice bran, or wheat germ.

- Ask them to smell jars of spices and herbs then pick their favorites.
- Go back and look at your interview sheets for favorite flavors or offer a taste test for sauces and dips like salsa, hummus, or yogurt.
- Try our tasty recipes, too!

Shapes and Do-dads

The more you can turn healthy eating into playtime, the more success you'll enjoy. Sometimes it just takes a minute to make a lunch special and appealing.

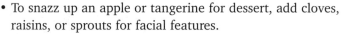

- To snazz up an apple or tangerine for dessert, add cloves, raisins, or sprouts for facial features.
- Use fancy toothpicks for mini-kabobs.
- Whip up some cheater chopsticks. Have your child try this at home first, and if it's fun, use it for some lunches. Wrap a rubber band around chopsticks from a restaurant and then wad a piece of paper or the original wrapper between the sticks. Works like fun tongs for most any age.
- Orange rind dragon teeth are great for brave young eaters.

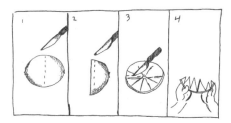

Toothpick and Dragon Teeth illustrations courtesy Paul McClendon, Age 12.

5. Cool looks—it's a fun thing

You can get a lot of mileage out of this tip. Kids respond to visual cues from their food. A cucumber can sit on a plate forever, but a cucumber-radish-asparagus *man* gets gobbled up in seconds. Ways to spiff it up:

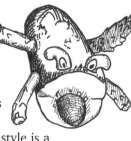

- Dip fruit in orange, lemon, or pineapple juice. This keeps them looking fresh and tasty all day long.
- For young children, cut food in bite-size pieces. Julienne style is a fancy term for very thinly sliced veggies like carrots.
- Offer nori or California rolls (see recipe on page 78) to introduce kids to the Japanese art of food presentation.
- Send lunch wrapped like a present, with card and a fun note in tow.
- Use snazzy paper muffin cups.
- Employ some lunchbox *feng shui*. Make the vegetable or fruit the centerpiece, using plenty of eye-appealing arrangement and flavor.

- Add a dash of sprinkles to a treat. Those little guys are kid magnets.
- Use a large glass or cookie cutters to cut out circles or make age appropriate appealing shapes for sandwiches.
- There are all kinds of shapes for pasta, and the sillier the better. Keep an eye out for something a little more interesting than elbow macaroni.
- On summer days when the lunchbox is up in the cupboard, fan out cheese and cuts of meat like the deli department trays for make-your-own cracker or bread sandwiches.
- Pack straws, the sillier the better.
- Arrange fruit or vegetables in rainbow order on nonfat cream cheese or hummus in a container: red, orange, yellow, green blue, purple
- Dazzle them with a flash of color by snazzing up bags and containers with stickers or magic marker art (tricks of the advertising trade).

The Rainbow Connection

Adding a little color, whether it's natural color or artificial*, gives a lunch pizzazz. Try the following additives to brighten a meal:

- Orange: beta carotene** (a small amount)
- Gold: turmeric, which is good with soups, salad dressings, and dips
- Yellow: edible dried flowers, such as chamomile, for a light yellow color
- Pink: beet juice (could grate or press to get a few drops of juice for pretty pink; or try the juice from canned beets)
- Blue: blueberries blended in a drink, yogurt, or nonfat cream cheese
- Green: lightly cooked kale blended with one cup water is great added to soup

 * Some kids react to artificial coloring. Check with your pediatrician about using supplements to add color to foods.

** Some studies have suggested that beta carotene may not be safe if your child has diabetes. Talk to your doctor and if you've been given the okay, ask for beta-carotene or mixed carotene supplements at a health food store. Solaray makes a mixed carotene called Food Carotene. Add a bit to cream cheese, frosting, or milk and you'll have a beautiful orange color plus the benefits of Vitamin A—antioxidant protection and vision support. Remember that it's best to get your nutrients from foods.

6. Educate to motivate

Knowledge is a powerful tool. We underestimate our kids sometimes and forget that they operate on reason just like adults (sometimes, much more often than adults). Kids need to understand that eating healthy is not just some arbitrary decision designed to punish. Plus, you can use experience to get your point across. Even very young children can connect the outcome of overeating junk food versus good food—good feeling. Ask your child to notice how they feel after eating certain foods from each side. They may not even notice this until you point it out. This puts more responsibility on them and helps take the nagging out of the picture.

Ask your librarian for children's books on healthy eating. There are tons of interesting stories that stress the importance of a healthy diet. We've also listed some kid-friendly books and educational websites in the resources section in the back of the book.

Picky Eaters

After junk food jealousy, this is your next biggest hurdle. Fortunately, Marie knows picky. As a child, she only ate two fruits and two vegetables. She tried her first orange at the tender age of 31. Now she gets to be the nutritionist in the family and battle the finicky taste buds. Her mother claims justice has been served at last.

Seven ways to encourage picky eaters
1. Don't force it.

- Offer just one new food at a time with an old favorite. Let your kids know if it will be salty, sour, savory, or sweet. Remember that texture and looks play a large part in taste.
- Diffuse power struggles with humor, not aggression.
- Use eye-appeal, like the Salad in a Green Pepper Boat with Cheese Sail pictured on page 30.
- Don't force a child to eat. Use simple, reasonable rules, like the at-least-one-bite-rule for trying new foods.
- Limit using unhealthy food as a reward. This sets a very bad trend of matching fatty or sugary treats with positive behavior. This is the wrong road to get started down.
- Don't expect your child to appreciate your efforts.
- Don't worry if your child goes through a phase of eating one thing. Continue offering a variety of foods; if they're hungry, they'll eat what you offer.

2. Involve the child in preparing food.

We love this advice and will keep giving it over and over. And there's no reason to stop in the kitchen, either. If you've got the space, plant a garden full of healthy vegetables and herbs. If you don't have the acreage, volunteer at someone else's vegetable patch. If kids are proud of meals they cook, imagine how proud they'll be of food they've grown and harvested themselves! Who could resist a vegetable that he or she had a part in creating?

3. Offer choices from a variety of different flavors and textures.

A great resource is the book, *One Bite Won't Kill You—More than 200 Recipes to Tempt Even the Pickiest Kids on Earth and The Rest of the Family Too*, by Ann Hodgman. It's packed with tasty alternatives.

Flavor is important for sure, but sometimes texture rules the day. Keep these texture tips in mind:

- Preserve the crunch! Pack the salad dressing and/or croutons separately or pack individual condiment packets found in fast food restaurants (McDonald's teamed up with Paul Newman's to produce nutritious single-serve natural salad dressings. You can buy packets without having to buy the salad. This is still a mega-portion, so ask your kid to use 1/2 the packet).
- Don't pack graham crackers with filling the night before.
- If a tomato is feeling squishy, leave it out.
- Place dry green pepper or something between bread slices and lettuce to stop the sog.
- Cut off bread crusts if always left uneaten. No guarantees here that the child still won't leave the edges!
- Send crunchers for munchers: baked chips, nuts, spiced nuts, tamari seeds, water chestnuts, crunchy veggies like jicama, carrots, cucumbers, radishes, red peppers, water chestnuts, and celery.

4. Use toppers to tone down (or boost) strong (or weak) flavors.

Sauces and dips can be a great way to make healthy foods with a strong flavor more palatable to finicky palates. Raw broccoli is a health food juggernaut, but the taste can be a little overpowering. Serve up a little melted cheese or diluted ranch dressing on the side and you've got a treat most kids will love.

5. A cauliflower by any other name...

A lot of picky eating starts when kids imagine they won't like a food before they've even tried it, and a lot of this could be tied to food names. Brussels sprouts have always been labeled the ultimate "ick" vegetable, so even if your picky eater hasn't actually eaten a Brussels sprout, they may have decided they don't like them. So try some new names to make things more interesting. Kids may yawn at regular green Jell-O, but shriek for Shrek Jell-O. Look at the way cereals are marketed to kids. Regular cold cereal suddenly becomes exciting and kid friendly with a little color and cartoon-shaped grains.

6. Set an example.

For some reason, parents, from time eternal, have believed their kids can't tell the difference between practicing and preaching. If anything, children learn almost everything from watching and way less from listening. Have you ever had a doctor tell you to lose weight, even though he's carrying around an extra sixty pounds himself? Pretty frustrating, isn't it? When you tell your kids to start chowing on vegetables while you wouldn't touch anything but French fries, you're doing the same thing. Your kids look to you for guidance, whether explicitly or not, for everything they do in their lives. Building their eating patterns is definitely on this list.

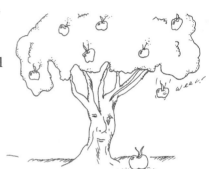

The apple doesn't fall far from the tree.

7. Be inventive, be sly.

• Hide apples in baked brownies by substituting applesauce for some of the butter.
• Sneak some cooked cauliflower into "smashed" (which is way cooler than mashed) potatoes.
• Boost tomato sauce or spaghetti sauce with raw carrots in the blender before cooking.
• Add ground fiber, such as bran or wheat germ.
• Liquefy steamed broccoli with broth or water and add to taco seasoning mix or spaghetti sauce.
• "Spruce up" Macaroni and Cheese with broccoli trees (get it? Spruce? Trees? Hey, we're trying our best here).

"Hey, Kiddo" Notes

Sometimes, just a little loving touch is all you need to give a healthy lunch something special, something that hints you care. Every kid is different. Some might be thrilled with a little pink note covered in balloons and teddy bears; others might be absolutely horrified. You know your kid best, so what you do is up to you. Following are some of the things that have worked for us.

- Love notes, like "Hey, Sunshine!" "Love You, Sugar Dumplin'," "Sending you a squeeeeze hug." (Caution! Know your kids' embarrassment threshold.)
- Riddles, jokes, tongue twisters, lines from mutually loved songs, limericks, or poems.
- Notes with a plan, such as "Let's go to the river after school," or "We'll go see Uncle Ernie when you get home." Other tactical maneuvers include trips to the playground, a stop by the bagel shop, a quick look at the bookstore, mystery snacks planted at home, meeting up with neighbors after school, or going camping for the weekend.
- For the kids horrified by the balloons and bears, secret coded messages are great, possibly hidden from classmates' views in a mutually agreed spot in the lunchbox. Color-coded quick option: blue means, "We'll do something under the blue sky," green means, "You're growing as fast as Jack's beanstalk!" red means, "I love you."

Lunchbox Architecture— Keeping the Hot Food Hot and the Cold Food Cold

Like flavor and texture, temperature plays a pretty big part in keeping lunchtime favorites tasty. Cold soup is always going to end up down the drain. To keep hot food hot, try the following:

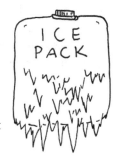

- Invest in a good thermos; they really work. Or place a cheaper thermos in a zip-top bag or a thermal bag (what deli chicken comes in) to help insulate and contain leaks. Even a paper bag will help.
- Pour boiling water into a thermos, put lid on top, and let it sit for a few minutes; empty and fill with food or drink.
- Wrap heated food in foil and then in a bag or bundle up in a small hand towel.

For keeping cold food cold, try these chilly techniques:

- Ice cubes in a leak-proof container will keep food cool.
- Look for cold packs in stores.
- Freeze juice or water in short, half-full water bottles for a dual-purpose drink.
- Freeze water in empty yogurt cups and then place upright in a twist-tie plastic bag for a homemade cold pack.

Ice Pack Illustration courtesy Anna McClendon, Age 10.

- Place frozen corn, peas, or berries in a small container for a refreshing side dish that keeps the rest of the lunch cold. (They will most likely be thawed by lunchtime.)
- Freeze yogurt cups or tubes for a cool dairy delight.

If you're worried about the safety of plastic containers, use plastics that have triangle recycling numbers 1, 2, 4, and 5. Avoid using microwave plastic products that don't clearly state "Safe for microwave use."

Divide and Conquer

Divided food containers are a lifesaver. They take up less space in the lunchbox and help keep dry things dry. For example, you can put salad dressing in one compartment and the salad in another—even croutons in a third compartment. Just remind your child to keep it level so the salad dressing doesn't escape.

Tell-Tale Sign—The Curse of the Uneaten Food Odor

Even with all of these brilliant ideas, you're gonna have some flops. And you know when a lunchtime experiment has gone wrong. The nose doesn't lie. Nothing reeks like a tuna sandwich left inside a lunchbox for an entire weekend.

Some schools have a policy that uneaten lunchbox food can't be thrown away, but must be returned home for feedback to parents. This is a fantastic way to see what works and what doesn't. You can't fine-tune your packing without honest feedback. If your school doesn't have such a policy, suggest it. And be sure to check your child's lunchbox.

If you're really curious, play detective and talk to school employees in the lunchroom who witness a lot of food slam-dunkin' into the trash cans. Make sure they know who your child is and ask them for information.

All in all though, remember to have a relaxed attitude about uneaten food and ask your child why they didn't like certain things instead of scolding them for letting it sit. If you've already got a good lunchbox relationship with your children, you cannot only ask how they liked lunch, you can brainstorm with them how to improve what they didn't like. "Too much mayonnaise" is easy to fix.

Chapter Five
Mom, I Can't Find the Tuna!
Creating a Kid-Friendly Kitchen

You may remember the hundred or so times we've encouraged getting kids involved with the lunch-making process. We can't help it; we just think it's a terrific idea. Not only does it promote healthier eating, but it also gives the family an excuse to be around one another, be creative, and just have fun.

When are kids ready to pack their own lunches? When they show an interest!

In this chapter, we go through some tips and techniques for organizing a kitchen everyone can use.

Organizing the Lunch-Making Area

Stash nonperishable foods on a lower cupboard or counter reachable by any kid interested in packing his or her own lunch. Put each kind of item in a separate labeled basket or box for easy food choices. A pull-out shelf works great in this situation, but if you don't have one, consider using a turntable or a tray that can be pulled out.

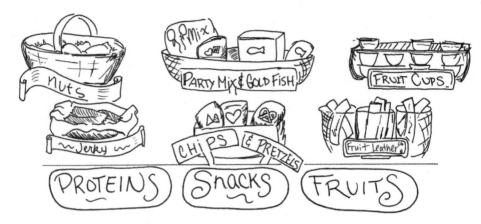

Non-refrigerated perishables (okay, breads) need to be assigned to a consistent spot out in the open and easily accessible. Out of sight, out of mind. Breads and bagels perched on top of the refrigerator will also mold faster.

Proper Precision

Cristy has been introducing her daughter to baking since she was three. It's amazing how accurate she was at measuring from the beginning, once mom modeled how to do it. She takes great pride in foods she has a hand in preparing. Cristy can't wait 'til she's big enough to reach the sink and help with the dishes afterward!

To give kids a leg-up packing a balanced lunch, post our handy dandy Lunchbox Blueprint (page 53) inside the kid-friendly pantry or nearby. Perhaps keep the same right-to-left or top-to-bottom order as the Blueprint: protein foods, then grains and cereals, dried and fresh fruits, and snacks or treats last. Labeling the cupboard with words or pictures for these food groups will help maintain order.

Finally, don't expect miracles. The skill of organizing is a life-long learning curve for some folks. And even the most organized kitchen isn't always going to have the young ones itching to whip up lunch. Be patient.

Ready for Rush Hour

Be sure to consider traffic patterns in your kitchen. If the kitchen is an interstate between rooms in your house, plan work areas carefully. You don't want to compete with frantic kids for room to pack. Open up some real estate with cupboard organizers. These are available for bags, plastic, foil wrap, and waxed paper. A nearby drawer works, too.

Container storage

It's amazing how quickly a cupboard of plastic containers can descend into complete anarchy, especially when you've got more than one set of hands in the mix. To keep things halfway organized, we keep one drawer for round containers and one for rectangular. Finding the right lid can become a time-consuming search and rescue mission. Lids will stack well in an organizer or simply on top of one another in a narrow box.

Countertops

Choose an area to reserve for lunch packing and keep knives, cutting board, etc., close by. If you have a set of canisters, use them to store frequently used lunch items. Marie's family keeps almonds in a canister near the blender since they use them in smoothies every morning.

Keep a filled fruit bowl near the lunch-packing station. Some families use a clear punch bowl for fruit so the fruits on the bottom aren't out-of-sight and forgotten. Besides, after years of being used every seventeen months or so, punch bowls often yearn for a purpose in life!

Refrigerator

Label the shelves and drawers in the fridge with words and/or icons so kids know where to find and replace items, such as condiments, cheese, yogurt, and leftovers. The refrigerator door may be the easiest place for kids to find things. That backbreaking shelf on the bottom of the door is just the right height for little lunch makers. Put stuff they use there!

Weekend jobs

Taking some time on weekends to organize can help save valuable minutes during the hectic pace of the weekdays. Divide regular or economy-size cans of baked beans, fruit, apple sauce, salad dressing, dips, and soy sauce into single-serving containers or bags and stack in the fridge.

For kids who need or want to go breadless, roll up deli meat (or deli meat and cheese), pack in sandwich bags, add 1/2 cup frozen vegetables, and store away in the freezer, ready for you or your child to pop into that lunchbox. No ice pack needed—thawed by lunchtime!

Making muffins, cookies, brownies, and other breads can be weekend family projects. Early experiences in the kitchen may set the tone for a lifetime attitude about cooking, so make this time fun and relaxing for your child. These are times to enjoy being elbow-deep in flour and to not worry so much about spills.

Chapter Six
What About Breakfast?

Grab-and-Go Grub for Breaking the Fast—
When They Have to Eat on the Run or Go Hungry

This *is* a lunch book, but we'd be a little remiss to ignore the importance of the first meal of the day. To boost brain-power, mood, and a healthy metabolism, eating a balanced breakfast helps kids soar in school. And this isn't just us talking; there are *a lot* of studies to back this up. Starting the day with a full belly also makes it less likely that kids will grab a snack with high calories later in the day.

> *Eat like a king for breakfast,*
> *A prince for lunch,*
> *And a pauper for supper.*
> **–Old English saying**

Morning Munchables

For some nutritious first-thing-fuel, here are some twists on old standbys and some new ideas to break that fast before school starts. The list covers everything from grab-and-go-grub to sit-and-savor breakfast:

- Banana and a handful of nuts (keep a stash of nuts in the car, if climate allows)
- Glass of milk or rice milk and a protein bar or homemade granola bar
- Peanut butter or nut butter on apple
- Two peanut butter and jelly sandwiches—one for breakfast, one for lunch (especially if there's some good lunchtime trading planned!)

- Near milkshakes (see box)
- Corn muffins with a little added ham, cheese, fiber, or protein
- In the cold cereal arena find inexpensive puffed grains with no added sugar and compliment nicely with some fresh or dried fruit (if the kids aren't ready to go cold turkey on the morning bowl of frosted sugar bombs, mix lower-sugar cereals with the sweet stuff now and faze them out over time)
- Cottage cheese and fruit
- Quick hot cereals or grains soaked overnight to cut down on the cooking time
- Pancakes with peanut butter (leftover pancakes zip back to life in the toaster)
- Quinoa flakes, millet, or leftover rice with maple flavoring, sweetener, pecans, and vanilla
- Eggs-in-a-Frame—Using a glass or cookie cutter, cut holes in a slice of bread, drop in an egg, and fry both sides. Or use a tall metal cookie cutter sprayed with oil to cut out shapes from scrambled eggs
- Green Eggs and Ham—just add spinach, kale, parsley, or cilantro
- Yogurt with fruit never fails
- Bagels with protein spreads, such as nut butters or seed butters
- Eggs—boiled, fried, omelet, or scrambled with cheese and veggies
- Overnight hot cereal made with whole kernel wheat or cracked wheat—heat water to boiling on the stove and pour over wheat, cover, and set overnight

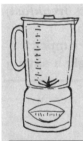

Near Milkshakes

Not quite milkshakes, but these doppelgangers will be close enough for rushed mornings.

Yogurt + berries with cereal for crunch
Milk + banana
Milk + fresh or frozen berries + a bit of sweetener

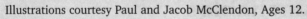

Illustrations courtesy Paul and Jacob McClendon, Ages 12.

More Morning Tips

Ideally, organize as much as you can the night before, rise early enough to get yourself ready, and then greet your kids with a smile (or at least not a growl).

- Oatmeal Shortcut #1: Grind oatmeal in a coffee grinder for faster cooking.
- Oatmeal Shortcut #2: Soak regular or steel-cut oats overnight. They'll cook in a fraction of the time in the morning. Follow directions on the container for amounts.

- Oatmeal Shortcut #3: Mix 1/2 cup quick oats with 1 cup milk or rice milk in medium mixing bowl and microwave for 2 minutes. Add cinnamon, nuts, or fruits.
- Nut butter toppings on pancakes or French toast up the protein, and apple-sauce topping is better than sugary syrup (though you could go half and half to ease the transition).

Drive-Thru Dilemma

Do you wait in line for ten minutes at the fast food joint for a bag of egg and cheese sandwiches and hash browns? Guess what, you just had time to make some much healthier oatmeal—and save a chunk of change.

Potential Stress-Buster for those Maniac Mondays

One reason parents are short on time in the morning is because getting the kids out the door can be like herding kittens. To keep things running smoothly, a single mother worked out this deal with her child: If her daughter was completely ready for school before a timer rang, they would have 10 minutes to roughhouse, read, or play a game before school. Not only did it get things organized in the morning, it gave them time together that they both enjoyed.

Make a checklist or picture list for your child. For example, the list could read:

- ☑ Dressed
- ☑ Breakfast
- ☑ Hair
- ☑ Teeth brushed
- ☑ Lunch packed
- ☑ Play time

Chapter Seven
This Isn't So Hard!

Handy Menu Rotation Charts and a Lunchbox-Packing Blueprint Guide to Keep the Lunch Packer on Track

Hopefully by now you've got a pretty good handle on what makes a healthy lunch. We've gone through a quick nutrition lecture, dropped some hints on kitchen organization, and revealed some insider info on the special touches that stave off lunch-boxer rebellions. Now we'll give you a quick look at how we've taken this information and used it to construct some healthy lunches. Feel free to use these examples to craft your own lunches (lunchbox plagiarism is A-okay) or simply use them for inspiration of your own. We'll start with our Rotation Menu Chart of sample meals for a whole month of munching. Use it as a guide to create a chart tailored to your family's preferences.

Rotation Menu Chart

Quick Fixes

These meals are a snap to throw together in the mornings. Some are made of interesting combinations lying around the kitchen, others take advantage of some quick recipes in Section 3. Either way, these are stress-free solutions to hectic mornings.

• Cold cereal packed with milk in a thermos • Baby carrots • Banana	• Cheese cubes or small slices • Crackers • Baby carrots • Apple	• Burrito • Tossed salad • Pomegranate
• Leftover bean and vegetable soup • Slice of cheese • Carrots and celery • Tamari almonds • Apple	• Cottage cheese with fruit • Radishes or Ants-on-a-Log • Granola Bar (p. 119)	• Canned vegetable soup • Whole-grain bread with butter • Favorite nuts • Tomato and lettuce with a favorite dressing • Pudding or apple
• Turkey or tempeh sandwich • Broccoli with ranch dressing • Homemade Fruit Leather (p. 92)	• Peanut butter and jelly sandwich • Cucumber with dip • Orange	• Tuna salad • Dill pickle • Celery with nonfat cream cheese • Grapes

Nine in about Nine Minutes

These tasty combinations take a little more time and rely on our recipes a bit more, but are still quick enough for Monday morning mania.

• Chili with grated cheese • Corn muffins • Veggie chunks with sauce • Yogurt with fruit	• Chinese Rolled Pancakes (p. 67) • Snow Peas with dip • Fruit slaw (p. 99) • Fortune cookie (p. 125)	• Deli Fajitas (p. 65) • Carrot sticks • Pineapple
• Mexican Pinwheels (p. 70) • Frozen corn on a toothpick • Kiwi or strawberries • Tapioca pudding	• Salmon and brown rice with soy sauce • Mixed carrots and peas • Sunflower seeds and raisins	• English Muffin Pizza (p. 91) • Sugar peas with dip • Kiwi
• Spicy Mac 'n' Cheese (p. 79) • Ants-on-a-log • Grapes	• Egg salad • Pickle on the side • Lettuce salad • Trail mix • Tangerine	• Rice with green chili sauce • Deviled eggs • Red pepper or jalapeño pepper • Yogurt with granola

Overnight Sensations

These lunches will take some preparation and planning, but believe us, the smiles and gratitude make the extra effort worthwhile.

• Tawny Scrawny Lion Soup (p. 84) • Veggie Pinwheels (p. 71) • Apple	• Overnight Bean Dip (p. 102) • Baked chips • Cucumber • Tangerine • Chocolate Chip Cookie (p. 114)	• Night-before pizza • Green peppers or carrots with dip • Canned mixed fruit
• Chicken Tortellini Salad (p. 85) • Baby carrots • Yogurt cup with fruit cubes • Blueberry muffin	• Laticia's Pollo (p. 83) • Spinach salad with cranberries and raspberry dressing • Brownie (p. 122)	• Native Pumpkin Soup (p. 74) • Fry bread • Celery (opt. salt shaker) • Homemade Fruit Leather (p. 92)

Lunchbox-Packing Blueprint Guide

If you're anything like us, this guide may very well become your best friend (in the kitchen anyway). Just having a visual mix-and-match list can simplify your morning tremendously, especially if you're still wiping the sleep from your eyes. We've listed a variety of choices for each of the four main components of lunch. Simply point a finger or throw a dart at any of foods from each section and you've got a lunch planned. It also doesn't hurt to copy this chart (or throw together one of your own), print it out, and post it in a conspicuous place in the kitchen. This makes it easier for interested kids to put together their own nutritious lunches (just make sure that you get one food from each column in there. The tendency to fill a box with four desserts can be a strong one).

Main Dish (Protein)	Fruit side	Vegetable Side	Snacks/Desserts
Can of baked beans	Fruit cups	Baby carrots	Homemade muffins
Crackers and nut butter	Applesauce	Peas	English muffins
Crackers and cheese	Apple	Corn	Pita bread
Yogurt	Banana	Broccoli	Party mix
Dinner leftovers	Pear	Cauliflower	Pudding cup
Cottage cheese	Berries	Vegetable mix	Fruit cup
Canned soup	Frozen berries	Bell pepper	Yogurt
Cup of noodles	Dried fruit	Celery	Any fruit or vegetable
Handful of nuts	100% juice boxes	Zucchini	Applesauce
Water-packed tuna	Raisins	Tomatoes	Crackers and cheese
Canned chicken	Grapes	Asparagus	Crackers and nut butter
Canned chili	Melon pieces	Water Chestnuts	Homemade cookies
English muffin with cheese	Homemade fruit leather	Jicama strips or cubes	Air-baked chips or popcorn
Bagel with cheese or meat	Orange or tangerine		Rice cakes
Hard-boiled eggs			Low-fat ranch dip
Jerky			Low-fat granola or cereal bars

Part Three: Go!

Wow, This Sounds Good:

Tasty Recipes for Healthy Lunches, Snacks, and Treats

Recipe Legend

To keep it simple and easy for all kinds of health plans and tastes, note the following recipe icons. These helpful symbols can give you an idea of what the recipe contains or how long it takes to prepare at a glance.

The Quick Fix Icon.
These recipes are simple and can be made in a snap. For rushed mornings or last minute inspiration, try these.

The Overnighter Icon.
These recipes usually call for a little more time and planning, so they're best prepared either the night before or when you have the time to "dance around the kitchen" and enjoy the process. These recipes are worth the effort because they: a) save you money (better spent on vacations or practical necessities), b) deliciously suit your family's tastes and health plans, and c) count as exercise if you use arm power instead of kitchen power tools!

The Gluten-Free Icon.
Gluten is a protein found in such grains as wheat, barley, rye, and oats, and is bad news for those with celiac disease. Common gluten-free flours include corn, rice, tapioca, and soy. (Buckwheat is wheat-less and gluten-less, believe it or not.) For severe gluten allergies consult the experts.

The Dairy-Free Icon.
As you can guess, dairy-free means just that—for those with dairy allergies or strict vegetarians.

Recipe List

Sandwiches, Salads, Soups, Casseroles, and Other Main Dishes

Fruit and Veggie Side Dishes and Snacks

Snacks and Desserts

Sandwiches, Salads, Soups, Casseroles, and Other Main Dishes

Asian Pasta Salad

Serving Size: 3/4 cup
Total Servings: 4
Prep Time: 20 minutes

Ingredients
1 cup corkscrew-shaped pasta, low-carb if possible (becomes 1 2/3 – 1 3/4 cups cooked)
2 oz snowpea pods, fresh (about 1/2 cup)
1 carrot (1/2 cup)
1/2 red bell pepper (about 1/2 cup)
1/2 jar (4 oz) baby corn, drained and rinsed
1/2 can (4 oz) mandarin oranges in juice, drained and juice saved

Asian Dressing
The juice from the 1/2 can of mandarin oranges
2 Tbsp light tamari soy sauce
2 Tbsp canola oil
1 tsp non-nutritive sweetener (or more to taste)
1/4 tsp ground ginger or 1/2 tsp ginger purée

Directions
1. Cook the pasta according to the directions on the box. Meanwhile, in a large bowl (large enough to hold all of the pasta and veggies) mix together the juice from the can of mandarin oranges, tamari, canola oil, non-nutritive sweetener, and ginger. Blend well (using a whisk is best). Taste and adjust seasoning if needed.

2. Once the pasta is done cooking, drain and rinse with cold water. Let it drain completely. Then add the pasta to the bowl with the dressing and toss.

3. Cut the pea pods into halves with a diagonal slice. Cut the carrot and the red bell pepper into 1 1/2-inch long, thin pieces. Slice the baby corn into halves cutting lengthwise. Place the veggies in with the pasta and toss well.

4. Add the mandarin oranges and lightly toss. Refrigerate. Divide salad into individual plastic serving containers for lunches.

Tasty Tip!
Try serving with tamari-roasted almonds on the side or mix in a few of those crunchy sesame sticks for more kid appeal.

Exchanges	Calories 150	Cholesterol 0 mg
1 Carbohydrate	Calories from Fat 70	Sodium 351 mg
1 Very Lean Meat	Total Fat 8 g	Total Carbohydrate 12 g
1 Fat	Saturated Fat 0.7 g	Dietary Fiber 4 g
	Polyunsaturated Fat 2.3 g	Sugars 6 g
	Monounsaturated Fat 4.3 g	Protein 9 g

Recipe courtesy of Lauri Ann Randolph, the award-winning author of Lauri's Low Carb Cookbook *and* Low Carb Creations from Lauri's Kitchen.

Butternut Soup w/ Ginger Butter

Serving Size: 1 cup, **Total Servings:** about 12
Prep time: 50 minutes
Baking Time: 45 minutes
Cooking time: 30 minutes

Ingredients
2 lb (about 4 cups) butternut squash
1/4 cup corn oil spread, tub
3/4 cup chopped onions
3/4 cup chopped celery
1/4 cup apple juice or applesauce
6 cups low-sodium vegetable or
  chicken broth
1 1/2 tsp vanilla extract

Directions
1. Cut squash lengthwise and remove seeds and strings. Place cut side down on greased baking sheet and bake for 45 minutes at 350°F. Let cool about 30 minutes.

2. Heat oil spread in large saucepan until melted. Scoop out squash pulp and add vegetables and cook over medium heat, stirring occasionally for about 5 minutes. Add apple juice to pan; cook 30 seconds.

3. Add broth. Heat to boiling. Reduce heat and simmer, covered, until squash is tender, about 25 minutes. Remove from heat; add vanilla.

4. Purée mixture in blender or food processor, half at a time. Serve in individual bowls.

Tasty Tip!
A thermos full of this soup goes great with corn muffins and a side fruit salad!

Add a small dollop of Ginger Butter!
1/4 cup non-hydrogenated oil spread
1 Tbsp grated fresh ginger, or
  2 tsp ginger paste, or
  1/2 tsp ground ginger
1 tsp maple syrup

Directions
1. Heat 1 Tbsp of oil spread in small skillet over medium heat. Add grated ginger. Cook 30 seconds.

2. Stir in ground ginger and maple syrup. Cook and stir about 30 seconds longer. Remove from heat. Let cool several minutes.

3. Combine remaining oil spread and ginger mixture in small bowls until smooth.

Nutrition information does not include Ginger Butter.

Exchanges	Calories 72	Cholesterol 0 mg
1/2 Starch	Calories from Fat 34	Sodium 226 mg
1/2 Fat	Total Fat 4 g	Total Carbohydrate 9 g
	Saturated Fat 0.7 g	Dietary Fiber 1 g
	Polyunsaturated Fat 1.2 g	Sugars 2 g
	Monounsaturated Fat 1.7 g	Protein 1 g

Baked Beans

Serving Size: 1/2 cup
Total Servings: 1
Prep time: 15 minutes
Cooking time: 1 hour

Ingredients
1 Tbsp vegetable oil
1/2 cup chopped onion
1 grated apple (peel left on if pesticide free)
1/2 tsp salt
1 tsp dry mustard powder
1/2 cup tomato paste
1/2 cup water
1 Tbsp molasses
4 cups canned vegetarian beans, such as pinto or Northern beans

Directions
1. Sauté oil and onion for 3 minutes. Add apple and cook covered over low heat for 5 minutes. Keep lid tight.
2. Mix remaining ingredients in a casserole pan that has a lid. Add in onion and apple mixture. Mix well.
3. Cover and bake for 45–60 minutes at 325°F. If you have a crock pot, use the time and setting recommended for canned beans.

Money-Saving Tip!
You can cook your own dried beans and not only save some cash, but have more control over the sodium content as well!

Groaner
Where do baby cows go to eat?
The calf-eteria!

Exchanges	Calories 113	Cholesterol 0 mg
1 1/2 Starch	Calories from Fat 15	Sodium 344 mg
	Total Fat 2 g	Total Carbohydrate 23 g
	Saturated Fat 0.2 g	Dietary Fiber 5 g
	Polyunsaturated Fat 0.6 g	Sugars 7 g
	Monounsaturated Fat 0.7 g	Protein 5 g

From The Best from the Family Heart Kitchens, a Guide to Low-Fat, Low-Salt Cooking, *Family Heart Study Nutrition Staff, Oregon Health Sciences University, 1981.*

Marie's Tangy Chicken and Peanut Butter Dipping Sauce

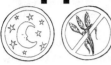

Serving Size: 3 Tbsp dip and 4 chicken strips
Total Servings: 8
Prep time: 15 minutes
Cooling time: 30 minutes

Ingredients
1 Tbsp olive oil
1 Tbsp sesame oil
1/2 cup diced red or mild onion
1 medium clove garlic, minced
1 1/2 tsp minced fresh gingerroot
1/4 tsp crushed red pepper flakes, if desired
2 Tbsp red wine vinegar or apple cider vinegar
1/4 cup fructose
1/2 tsp molasses
2 Tbsp reduced-sodium soy sauce or tamari (wheat-free if desired)
1/2 cup smooth peanut butter
1/4 cup mild salsa
2 tsp freshly squeezed lime juice
4 cups cooked skinless chicken breast strips

Directions
1. In a 10-inch skillet, over medium heat, cook oils, red onion, garlic, ginger root, and red pepper for 10 minutes, or until onion is softened. Beat or whisk in vinegar, fructose, molasses, soy sauce, peanut butter, salsa, and lime juice; cook one more minute. Cool before packing, especially when plastic containers are used.
2. If this thickens too much, wait until mixture cools and add a bit of water. Serve with vegetables or whole-grain crackers. For hesitant first-timers, the fun dipping stick may help.

Makes a Delicious Dressing, Too!
To transform this dip into a great-tasting salad dressing, thin the cooled sauce with a little water or half water and half rice |vinegar. Pour over 4 oz cold, cooked, thinly sliced beef or chicken, 1/2 cup chopped fresh baby bok choy or spinach, and 1/4 cup grated carrots and/or radishes for a main dish salad.

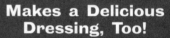

Exchanges	Calories 275	Cholesterol 60 mg
1 Carbohydrate	Calories from Fat 125	Sodium 277 mg
3 Lean Meat	**Total Fat** 14 g	**Total Carbohydrate** 11 g
1 Fat	Saturated Fat 2.2 g	Dietary Fiber 1 g
	Polyunsaturated Fat 3.4	Sugars 8 g
	Monounsaturated Fat 6.8	**Protein** 26 g

Deli Fajita

Serving size: 1 fajita sandwich
Total Servings: 1
Prep time: 5 minutes

Ingredients
1 6-inch flour tortilla
2 oz (2 slices) thinly sliced deli
  meats, such as ham, turkey, pastra-
  mi, roast beef, etc.
1/4 cup finely shredded lettuce
1/4 cup diced tomato
1 1/2 Tbsp grated reduced-fat sharp
  cheddar, American, Jack, or Colby
1 Tbsp reduced-fat ranch dressing

Directions
1. Layer on tortilla in the following
   order: meat, lettuce, tomatoes,
   cheese, and dressing.
2. Roll up and eat!

Groaner
What green dip do Mexican
ducks eat at piñata parties?

Quack-amole!

Appetizing Alternatives

- Cut a slice of pita bread (pocket
  bread) in half and fill cavity with
  the ingredients for some Middle
  Eastern flair.

- Try mixing 1/2 tsp tamari with 1
  Tbsp low-fat mayonnaise dressing
  for an Oriental twist.

- Try turkey with provolone and use
  low-fat, herb-and-garlic-flavored
  cheese spread instead of ranch
  dressing. Substitute some favorite
  greens for the lettuce.

Exchanges	Calories 239	Cholesterol 49 mg
1 Starch	Calories from Fat 64	Sodium 655 mg
1 Vegetable	Total Fat 7 g	Total Carbohydrate 23 g
2 Lean Meat	Saturated Fat 2.4 g	Dietary Fiber 2 g
1/2 Fat	Polyunsaturated Fat 1.1 g	Sugars 4 g
	Monounsaturated Fat 2.6 g	Protein 19 g

Fruity Pasta Salad with Ham

Serving Size: 1 cup
Total Servings: 4
Prep time: 10 minutes
Chilling time: 2 hours

Ingredients
1/3 cup plain low-fat yogurt or
   soy yogurt
1/4 cup 1% milk
1/3 cup fat-free mayonnaise
2 cups cooked rotini pasta
1/2 cup seedless green or
   red grape halves
1/2 lb fully cooked extra lean, lower-
   sodium ham, cut into
   1/2 inch cubes (about 1 1/2 cups)
1 can (8 oz) pineapple tidbits,
   drained
1/2 cup grated carrots
1/2 cup diced celery

Directions
1. Stir yogurt and milk into
   mayonnaise and add to pasta.

2. Stir in remaining ingredients. Chill at
   least 2 hours.

Sneak Attack
This recipe is a great way to sneak
fruit and veggies into lunch!

Exchanges	Calories 251	Cholesterol 26 mg
2 Starch	Calories from Fat 19	Sodium 614 mg
1/2 Fruit	Total Fat 2 g	Total Carbohydrate 42 g
1 Vegetable	Saturated Fat 0.8 g	Dietary Fiber 2 g
1 Very Lean Meat	Polyunsaturated Fat 0.5 g	Sugars 16 g
	Monounsaturated Fat 0.6 g	Protein 16 g

Easy Chinese Rolled Pancakes

Serving Size: 1 pancake
Total Servings: 1
Prep time: 12 minutes

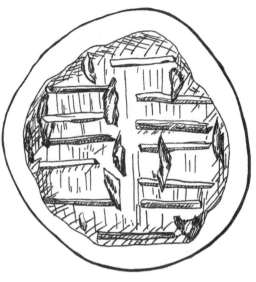

Ingredients
1 6-inch flour tortilla
1 tsp Hoisin sauce (see sidebar)
1/4 cup shredded cooked chicken, turkey, or pork (low-salt deli meat is okay)
1/4 cup (6 strips) cucumber or carrots, sliced into 2-inch long thin strips
1/4 cup (6 strips) celery, sliced into 2-inch long thin strips

Directions
1. Warm up tortilla in microwave oven, if desired.
2. Spread Hoisin sauce over half of tortilla. Arrange strips of meat and vegetables over sauce. Roll up like a burrito and enjoy!

If your grocer thinks Hoisin is a province in Thailand...

Hoisin is a Chinese sauce usually found in the Oriental section of the grocery store, but there's a chance your local store may not carry it. If not, substitute Chinese Plum Sauce, which is more readily available. If you can't find either, create your own sauce by combining plum, apricot, or pineapple-apricot jam with some reduced-sodium soy sauce and catsup (or salsa). The sauce should be slightly sweet-sour and salty. Other vegetables can be added, such as crunchy jicama strips or blanched bean sprouts.

Exchanges	Calories 171	Cholesterol 30 mg
1 Starch	Calories from Fat 31	Sodium 298 mg
1 Vegetable	**Total Fat** 3 g	**Total Carbohydrate** 20 g
1 Lean Meat	Saturated Fat 0.9 g	Dietary Fiber 2 g
	Polyunsaturated Fat 0.6 g	Sugars 3 g
	Monounsaturated Fat 1.6 g	**Protein** 14 g

Adapted from a recipe by Sandy Kinro.

1-2-3 Shrimp Party Plate

Serving Size: 1/2 cup with 6 non-gluten crackers
Total Servings: 1
Prep time: 5 nanoseconds
(with magic wand; 5 minutes without)

Ingredients
1/4 cup fat-free cream cheese
2 Tbsp salsa
2 Tbsp mashed canned, de-veined tiny shrimp, rinsed; or drained water-packed tuna

Directions
1. Place a sheet of wax paper on the bottom of a round container with a tight-fitting lid. Spread cream cheese thinly over the paper, like you are buttering bread (a back of a spoon works well).
2. Spread salsa over cream cheese.
3. Sprinkle with shrimp or tuna. Cover.
4. Pack sturdy crackers separately for dipping at lunch. Don't forget an ice pack!

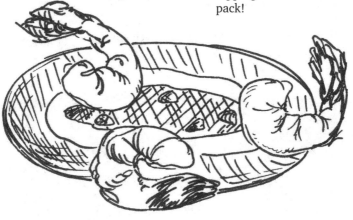

Exchanges
1 1/2 Starch
1 Lean Meat

Calories 197
    Calories from Fat 31
Total Fat 3 g
    Saturated Fat 0.2 g
    Polyunsaturated Fat 0.9 g
    Monounsaturated Fat 0.6 g

Cholesterol 36 mg
Sodium 540 mg
Total Carbohydrate 25 g
    Dietary Fiber 3 g
    Sugars 7 g
Protein 17 g

Purple People-Eaten Dip

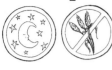

Serving Size: 1/2 cup dip, 1/2 hardboiled egg, 1/2 slice pita bread, **Total Servings:** 4
Prep time: 15 minutes
Baking time: 50–60 minutes
Chilling time: 2 hours or overnight

Ingredients
1 large eggplant (1 1/2 pounds)
2 cloves garlic, minced
2 Tbsp olive oil
2 Tbsp vinegar
1/2 tsp salt
1/2 tsp pepper
2 Tbsp chopped parsley
2 hardboiled eggs, sliced
1 medium tomato, cut into wedges, or 4 Tbsp sun-dried tomato pieces, chopped, and, if packed in oil, patted to remove excess oil
1/2 slice pita bread

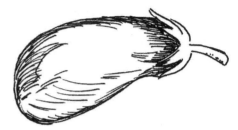

Directions
1. Pierce the eggplant several times with a fork. Bake at 350°F for 50–60 minutes, or until tender.

2. Remove skin while warm, and mash with a wooden spoon. Add the garlic, olive oil, vinegar, salt, pepper, and parsley. Chill 2 hours or overnight.

3. For lunch, scoop about 1/2 cup into a lunch container. If possible, place sliced hard-boiled egg and tomato slices (or sun-dried tomatoes) around edge of dip inside container. Or pack separately. Include pita bread.

Exchanges	Calories 245	Cholesterol 106 mg
1 Starch	Calories from Fat 97	Sodium 561 mg
3 Vegetable	**Total Fat** 11 g	**Total Carbohydrate** 32 g
2 Fat	Saturated Fat 1.9 g	Dietary Fiber 5 g
	Polyunsaturated Fat 1.3 g	Sugars 7 g
	Monounsaturated Fat 6.5 g	**Protein** 8 g

Mexican Pinwheels

Serving Size: 1 tortilla roll, sliced into pinwheels
Total Servings: 1
Prep time: 15 minutes
Chilling time: 2 hours

Ingredients
2 Tbsp canned fat-free refried beans
1 10-inch tortilla
2 Tbsp diced tomato
2 Tbsp drained cooked corn, cooled
1 Tbsp reduced-fat sharp cheddar (optional)
1/2 Tbsp finely chopped cilantro (optional)
2 Tbsp mashed avocado
1 Tbsp fat-free sour cream
2 Tbsp salsa

Directions
1. Spread the refried beans on the tortilla.

2. Sprinkle tomato, corn, and if desired, cheese and cilantro onto refried beans.

3. Mix avocado, sour cream, and salsa. Spread on top.

4. Roll up, chill for at least 2 hours. Slice into 1-inch pinwheels.

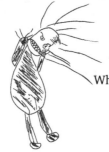

Groaner
What do monsters love to order at Mexican restaurants?
Re-fright beans.

Illustration courtesy Scott McClendon, Age 8.

Nutrition information does not include optional ingredients.

Exchanges	Calories 338	Cholesterol 1 mg
3 1/2 Starch	Calories from Fat 84	Sodium 565 mg
1 1/2 Fat	**Total Fat** 9 g	**Total Carbohydrate** 54 g
	Saturated Fat 1.9 g	Dietary Fiber 6 g
	Polyunsaturated Fat 1.4 g	Sugars 5 g
	Monounsaturated Fat 5.3 g	**Protein** 10 g

Veggie Pinwheels

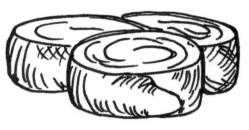

Serving Size: 1 tortilla roll, sliced into pinwheels
Total Servings: 1
Prep time: 15 minutes
Chilling time: 2 hours

Ingredients
1 Tbsp fat-free cream cheese
1 1/2 tsp fat-free ranch dressing
1 10-inch wheat tortilla
2 Tbsp finely chopped fresh
   broccoli, cooked or raw (or 1-1/2
   cups packaged broccoli slaw,
   finely processed)
2 Tbsp finely shredded carrots
Optional: one or two of the
   following:
- 1 1/2 tsp sunflower seeds,
- 1 Tbsp finely chopped sun-dried
  tomatoes packed in oil and
  patted with a paper towel to
  absorb oil,
- 1 1/2 tsp golden raisins,
- 1 Tbsp finely chopped water
  chestnuts or jicama, or
- 1 Tbsp mango chutney.

Directions
1. Stir ranch dressing into cream cheese. Spread mixture to within 1/4 inch of entire edge of tortilla.

2. In small bowl, mix broccoli, carrots, and any optional ingredients.

Sprinkle a thin layer of veggie mixture on top of the tortilla to within 1/4 inch of edge. Roll up and pin edge with toothpicks. Chill at least 2 hours. Slice into pinwheels one-inch thick.

Nutrition information does not include optional ingredients.

Exchanges	Calories 274	Cholesterol 1 mg
3 Starch	Calories from Fat 45	**Sodium** 521 mg
1/2 Fat	**Total Fat** 5 g	**Total Carbohydrate** 49 g
	Saturated Fat 1.2 g	Dietary Fiber 3 g
	Polyunsaturated Fat 0.8 g	Sugars 4 g
	Monounsaturated Fat 2.6 g	**Protein** 8 g

Gluten-Free Pizza

Serving Size: 1 slice
Total Servings: 6
Prep time: 30 minutes
Baking time: 30 minutes

Ingredients

Pizza Sauce
1 can (8 oz) tomato sauce
1/2 tsp dried oregano leaves
1/2 tsp dried basil leaves
1/2 tsp crushed dried rosemary
1/2 tsp fennel seeds
1/4 tsp garlic powder
2 tsp sugar
1/2 tsp salt

Crust
1 Tbsp dry yeast
2/3 cup brown rice flour or
    garbanzo/fava bean flour
1/2 cup tapioca flour
2 tsp xanthan gum
1/2 tsp salt
1 tsp unflavored gelatin powder
    (Knox)
1 tsp Italian herb seasoning
2/3 cup warm nonfat milk (110°F)
1/2 tsp sugar or honey
1 tsp olive oil
1 tsp cider vinegar
Extra rice flour for sprinkling

Toppings of your choice

Directions

Sauce

Combine all ingredients in small saucepan and bring to boil over medium heat. Reduce heat to low and simmer for 15 minutes while pizza crust is being assembled. Makes about 1 cup.

Crust

1. Preheat oven to 425°F. In medium mixing bowl using regular beaters (not dough hooks), blend the yeast, flours, xanthan gum, salt, gelatin powder, and Italian seasoning on low speed. Add warm milk, sugar, oil, and vinegar.

2. Beat on high speed for 2 minutes. (If the mixer bounces around the bowl, the dough is too stiff. Add water if necessary, one tablespoon at a time, until dough does not resist beaters.) The dough will resemble soft bread dough. (You may also mix in bread machine on dough setting.)

3. Put mixture on lightly greased 12-inch pizza pan. Liberally sprinkle rice flour onto dough. Press dough into pan, continuing to sprinkle dough with flour to prevent sticking to your hands. Make edges thicker to hold the toppings.

4. Bake pizza crust for 10 minutes. Remove from oven. Top pizza crust with sauce and your preferred toppings. Bake for another 20–25 minutes or until top is nicely browned.

Now Everyone Can Enjoy Pizza

Some of the ingredients may be a little hard to find, but this pizza is tailor-made for those who have to avoid recipes with gluten. Now the whole family can dig in!

Nutrition information is for crust and sauce only.

Exchanges	Calories 160	Cholesterol 1 mg
2 Starch	Calories from Fat 14	Sodium 634 mg
	Total Fat 2 g	Total Carbohydrate 34 g
	Saturated Fat 0.3 g	Dietary Fiber 3 g
	Polyunsaturated Fat 0.3 g	Sugars 5 g
	Monounsaturated Fat 0.9 g	Protein 4 g

Reprinted with permission from Gluten-Free 101: Easy, Basic Dishes without Wheat, *by Carol Fenster, PhD.*

Native Pumpkin Soup

Serving Size: 1 cup
Total Servings: 6
Prep time: 30 minutes
Cooking time: about 30 minutes

Ingredients
1 can (1 lb 13 oz) canned pumpkin
1 quart 1% milk
1 Tbsp butter
2 Tbsp honey
2 Tbsp maple syrup or light brown
   sugar
1/2 tsp powdered marjoram
dash white pepper
1/4 tsp cinnamon
1/4 tsp mace
1 tsp salt
juice of 1 orange

Directions
1. Heat pumpkin, milk, butter, and honey slowly together in a large saucepan, stirring.

2. Combine maple syrup, marjoram, pepper, cinnamon, mace, and salt. Stir into pumpkin mixture. Heat slowly, stirring constantly, until bubbles appear, but don't let it boil; about 20 minutes.

3. Add the orange juice, a little at a time. Serve hot.

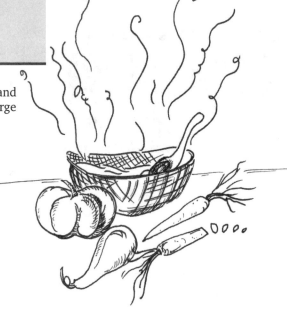

Exchanges	Calories 178	Cholesterol 13 mg
2 Carbohydrate	Calories from Fat 35	Sodium 490 mg
1/2 Fat	Total Fat 4 g	Total Carbohydrate 31 g
	Saturated Fat 2.5 g	Dietary Fiber 4 g
	Polyunsaturated Fat 0.2 g	Sugars 24 g
	Monounsaturated Fat 1 g	Protein 7 g

Turkey Lurkey Jerky

Serving Size: 1/4 recipe
Total Servings: 4
Prep time: 25 min
Baking time: 3–5 hours

Ingredients
1 lb boned and skinned turkey breast or tenderloins
1 Tbsp salt
1/2 cup water
1 1/2 Tbsp brown sugar
2 cloves garlic, minced, or pressed, or 1/4 tsp garlic powder
1/2 small onion, minced, or 1/2 tsp onion powder
1 tsp black or white pepper
1/2 tsp liquid smoke or wheat-free soy sauce
1/2 tsp ginger purée

Directions
1. Rinse meat and pat dry with paper towel. Remove fat and connective tissue. At this point, you may freeze meat about 15 minutes to make it firm for slicing. Cut into 1/2-inch thick slices. Cut breast with or against the grain and tenderloins lengthwise.

2. In a large bowl, stir together salt, water, brown sugar, garlic, onion, pepper, liquid smoke, and ginger purée. Add turkey and mix well. Cover and chill at least 1 hour or up to 24 hours.

3. Coat metal racks to cover a 10 x 15-inch baking pan with nonstick cooking spray.

4. Lift turkey strips from liquid, shake off excess, and lay strips close together, but not overlapping, on racks.

5. Preheat oven to 200°F. Place pan on center rack; prop door open about 2 inches. Dry until a cool (out of oven about 5 minutes) piece of jerky cracks and bends, about 3–5 hours.

6. Let jerky cool on racks, then remove. Serve, or store in airtight containers in a cool, dry place up to 3 weeks, in the refrigerator up to 4 months, or longer in freezer. Makes about 7 oz.

Tasty Tip!
For less saltiness, rinse strips and pat them dry before starting the drying process.

Exchanges	Calories 91	Cholesterol 54 mg
3 Very Lean Meat	Calories from Fat 4	Sodium 470 mg
	Total Fat 0 g	**Total Carbohydrate** 1 g
	Saturated Fat 0 g	Dietary Fiber 0 g
	Polyunsaturated Fat 0 g	Sugars 1 g
	Monounsaturated Fat 0 g	**Protein** 19 g

(Sort of) Ramen Nachos

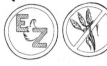

Serving Size: 3/4 cup
Total Servings: 3
Prep time: 10 minutes
Cooking Time: 3 minutes

Ingredients
1 package (3 oz) rice noodles, broken up
3 Tbsp reduced-fat grated cheddar cheese
1 cup canned chili
1 cup crushed baked corn chips
Optional: plain yogurt or sour cream and chopped green onion

Directions
1. Cook noodles in water according to package directions and drain. Add and stir warm noodles, cheese, and chili until cheese is melted.
2. Pack in thermos and add optional yogurt (or sour cream) and green onions.
3. Pack whole or crushed chips separately to keep crisp.

Gluten-Free Alert

Some pre-shredded cheeses are convenient, but have added flour, usually a gluten flour, to prevent caking.

Schoolyard Crush

Our kids enjoy crushing the chips over these nachos before eating, but digging in with whole chips means no need for forks or spoons!

Nutrition information does not include optional ingredients.

Exchanges	Calories 263	Cholesterol 48 mg
3 Starch	Calories from Fat 41	Sodium 537 mg
1/2 Fat	Total Fat 5 g	Total Carbohydrate 44 g
	Saturated Fat 1.8 g	Dietary Fiber 4 g
	Polyunsaturated Fat 0.6 g	Sugars 3 g
	Monounsaturated Fat 1.7 g	Protein 12 g

Recipe adapted for children on low-fat food plans from the book 101 Things to Do With Ramen Noodles, *by Toni Patrick.*

Paul's Savory Steak Soup

Serving Size: 1 cup
Total Servings: 10
Prep time: 30 minutes
Cooking time: 1 hour, 20 minutes

Ingredients

1 lb round steak, chopped into 1/2-inch cubes, or lean hamburger
1 medium onion, finely chopped (about 1 cup)
2 carrots, finely chopped (about 1 cup)
3 sticks celery, finely chopped (1-1/2 cups)
1 Tbsp butter
1/3 cup whole-wheat or barley flour or non-gluten thickener
1 1/2 cups canned, diced tomatoes
1 quart 99% fat-free beef stock
Salt and pepper to taste
1 tsp seasoned salt
2 tsp Worcestershire sauce
1/2 cup low-fat plain yogurt

Directions

1. Braise meat and onions in large pot. Add rest of vegetables, butter, and flour. Mix well and cook for 10 minutes. Add tomatoes, beef stock, and all spices; simmer for about 1 hour, stirring frequently.

2. Add yogurt the last 5 minutes before removing from heat. If mixture is too thick, add more beef stock and adjust seasoning.

Slow and Steady

This soup can also be slow cooked in a crock pot for 8–10 hours. Just braise the meat beforehand and warm the yogurt before adding in. This soup also freezes well.

Exchanges	Calories 103	Cholesterol 26 mg
2 Vegetable	Calories from Fat 29	Sodium 470 mg
1 Lean Meat	Total Fat 3 g	Total Carbohydrate 9 g
	Saturated Fat 1.4 g	Dietary Fiber 2 g
	Polyunsaturated Fat 0.2 g	Sugars 4 g
	Monounsaturated Fat 1.2 g	Protein 10 g

Nori Rolls
(aka, California Rolls)

Serving Size: 1 roll
Total Servings: 4
Prep time: 12 minutes

Ingredients
4 nori sheets (the McClendon kids
   like Eden's Sushi Nori)
2 cups sweet brown rice or sushi rice
1/2 cup diced cucumber
1/2 cup diced carrot
1/2 medium avocado sliced thin
1/2 cup greens: lettuce, cabbage, etc.
Optional: tofu, peppers, ginger slices,
   or ginger puree

Directions
1. Cook rice according to package directions. Place rice and all other ingredients inside the nori sheet closer to the end away from the spread.

2. Roll the nori sheet over the rice and vegetables. Dampen the end with water or ginger puree to seal.

3. Slice in 1-inch lengths or eat it like a burrito.

Dead Ocean Grass Probably Isn't Wise Either
You may want to call the wrapping sheets nori or California roll paper instead of seaweed to cut down on the hate-it-before-they-try-it factor.

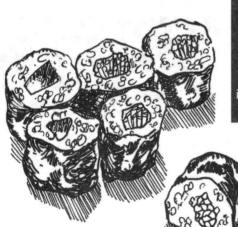

Nutrition information does not include optional ingredients.

Exchanges	Calories 157	Cholesterol 0 mg
1 1/2 Starch	Calories from Fat 37	Sodium 23 mg
1 Vegetable	Total Fat 4 g	Total Carbohydrate 26 g
1/2 Fat	Saturated Fat 0.7 g	Dietary Fiber 3 g
	Polyunsaturated Fat 0.8 g	Sugars 2 g
	Monounsaturated Fat 2.2 g	Protein 4 g

Spicy Mac 'n' Cheese with Broccoli

 Serving Size: 2/3 cup
Total Servings: 6
Prep time: 15 minutes

Ingredients
1 cup low-carb or regular elbow macaroni
1 1/2 cups broccoli, chopped (fresh or frozen)
1/2 cup Tostitos Salsa Con Queso

Directions
1. Cook pasta according to directions over medium high heat for the minimum cooking time indicated on the box. For example, if the box says to cook for 8 to 10 minutes, then cook for only 8 minutes.

2. Add chopped broccoli during last 2 minutes of cooking time. If broccoli is frozen, then add it for just the last 1 minute.

3. Drain pasta well and return it to cooking pot and reduce heat to medium low. Add the Tostitos cheese sauce, stir, and heat through (about 1 minute). Store in a wide-mouth thermos to keep hot.

Sneak Attack
Having trouble getting your kids to eat broccoli? This spicy cheese sauce will make them ask for more.

Appetizing Alternative
Tostitos Salsa Con Queso is the medium-spicy cheese sauce that you find in the snack aisle of the grocery store. Naturally, you can use any brand that you like. For extra spicy flavor, add a dash of Tabasco sauce or chili powder when you add the cheese sauce.

Nutrition information is for regular macaroni.

Exchanges	Calories 97	Cholesterol 0 mg
1 Carb	Calories from Fat 21	Sodium 193 mg
1/2 Fat	Total Fat 2 g	Total Carbohydrate 15 g
	Saturated Fat 1 g	Dietary Fiber 1 g
	Polyunsaturated Fat 0.3 g	Sugars 2 g
	Monounsaturated Fat 0.6 g	Protein 3 g

Recipe is courtesy of Lauri Ann Randolph, the award-winning author of Lauri's Low Carb Cookbook *and* Low Carb Creations from Lauri's Kitchen.

Marinated Vegetable Filling for Sandwiches

Serving Size: 1/2 cup
Total Servings: 8
Prep time: 10 minutes with food processor

Ingredients
4 cups raw vegetables (onions, bell peppers, zucchini, parsnips, cucumbers, carrots, etc.)
1/4 cup balsamic vinegar
1 Tbsp olive oil
salt and pepper to taste

5 a Day
A great way to up those daily vegetable servings per day! This one also keeps well, so make as much as you want.

Directions
Slice all vegetables thinly. Toss with oil, vinegar, and seasonings. Cover and marinate in the fridge for several hours or overnight.

Exchanges
1 Vegetable

Calories 33
Calories from Fat 16
Total Fat 2 g
Saturated Fat 0.2 g
Polyunsaturated Fat 0.2 g
Monounsaturated Fat 1.2 g

Cholesterol 0 mg
Sodium 13 mg
Total Carbohydrate 5 g
Dietary Fiber 1 g
Sugars 2 g
Protein 1 g

Overnight Layered Salad

Serving Size: 1 cup
Total Servings: 10
Prep time: 30 minutes

Ingredients
1/2 a head (3 cups) lettuce of your choice
5 stalks (2 cups) chopped celery
1/4 cup green bell pepper, chopped, or one small cucumber, chopped
1 small sweet onion (1/2 cup), or 2 green onions (include green tops), finely chopped
2 carrots (1 cup) grated or chopped
1 package (10 oz) frozen peas, thawed
1 cup shredded reduced-fat sharp cheddar
1 1/2 cups fat-free mayonnaise or salad dressing (check for gluten and low-sugar, if needed)
Optional: bacon bits, sunflower seeds, chopped almonds, chopped hard-cooked egg, or chopped sun-dried tomatoes

Directions
1. Layer first 7 ingredients in four 4 x 5-inch plastic containers (for easy packing), starting with lettuce and working up to the cheese.

2. Spread top with 1/2-inch layer of fat-free mayonnaise or salad dressing.

3. Cover with plastic wrap and chill in refrigerator overnight.

4. If desired, sprinkle optional ingredients on top at serving time.

Tasty Tip!
This recipe gets better with time, so for increased flavor, make it up to a day before packing it into lunchboxes. Of course, you can serve it right away if you want. Very colorful when placed in a clear container.

Nutrition information does not include optional ingredients.

Exchanges	Calories 82	Cholesterol 6 mg
1 Carbohydrate	Calories from Fat 18	**Sodium** 375 mg
	Total Fat 2 g	**Total Carbohydrate** 12 g
	Saturated Fat 1.1 g	Dietary Fiber 2 g
	Polyunsaturated Fat 0.1 g	Sugars 5 g
	Monounsaturated Fat 0.5 g	**Protein** 4 g

Crunchy Munchy Lunchy Chicken

Serving Size: 1 drumstick, 2 wings, 1 thigh, or 1/2 breast
Total Servings: 7
Prep time: 25 minutes
Baking time: 40 minutes

Ingredients
1 chicken (3 lb), cut up
1 cup low-fat buttermilk
1 cup flour
  (whole grain, if you prefer)
1–2 tsp paprika or red pepper flakes,
  or 1/2 tsp ground rosemary
1 tsp seasoned salt
pepper to taste
6 oz chopped pecans

2. Put flour mixture into a sturdy plastic bag; add 2 pieces of chicken at a time to bag and shake over the sink. Dip into buttermilk again, then roll and press chicken into pecans.

3. Bake for 20 minutes. Using long fork or tongs with oven mitt on hand, turn the chicken and bake for 20 minutes longer or until juice runs clear when stuck with a knife.

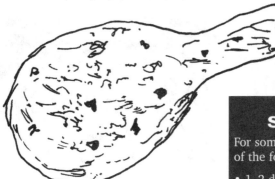

Directions
1. Preheat oven to 400°F. Put buttermilk into a large bowl and soak chicken pieces in buttermilk for about 5 minutes.

Spicy Variations

For some spicy alternatives, add one of the following to the buttermilk:

• 1–2 drops Tabasco OR

• 3–4 sprigs finely chopped fresh oregano OR

• 2 Tbsp spicy brown mustard

Exchanges
1 Starch
3 Lean Meat
1 1/2 Fat

Calories 289
  Calories from Fat 155
Total Fat 17 g
  Saturated Fat 2.4 g
  Polyunsaturated Fat 4.5 g
  Monounsaturated Fat 8.9 g

Cholesterol 57 mg
Sodium 245 mg
Total Carbohydrate 13 g
  Dietary Fiber 3 g
  Sugars 2 g
Protein 22 g

Laticia's Pozole de Pollo (Chicken Hominy Thick Stew)

Serving Size: 1 cup
Servings: 6
Prep time: 10 minutes
Cooking time: 15 minutes

Ingredients

3 cups cooked chicken
1 can (16 oz) white hominy or corn
3/4 cup onion, chopped
1/4 tsp oregano
1/2 cup fresh cilantro or parsley
2 cloves pressed garlic
salt to taste
4 dried colorful dried red chili peppers (pasilla, ancho), finely chopped, or 1/2 cup salsa

Directions

1. Brown onions in large frying pan.
2. Add other ingredients except salsa and cook on medium-high about 10 minutes.
3. Add salsa to taste and heat through, about 5 minutes. Cook most of the water out.
4. Serve with rice or beans. Best when kept warm in thermos, but can be eaten cold.

Direct Quote

"Mom, can we have that again?"

—Jacob McClendon

Exchanges	Calories 203	Cholesterol 62 mg
1 Starch	Calories from Fat 53	Sodium 276 mg
2 Lean Meat	Total Fat 6 g	Total Carbohydrate 14 g
	Saturated Fat 1.5 g	Dietary Fiber 2 g
	Polyunsaturated Fat 1.5 g	Sugars 3 g
	Monounsaturated Fat 2.0 g	Protein 22 g

Recipe courtesy of Laticia Cardenas.

Tawny Scrawny Lion Carrot Soup

Serving Size: 1 cup
Total Servings: 8
Prep time: 10 minutes
Cooking time: 40 minutes

Ingredients

2 lb carrots
4 cups fat-free 60% less vegetarian broth
1/2 tsp salt
1 tsp ginger paste
1 Tbsp butter
1 cup chopped red or yellow onion
1–2 small cloves garlic, pressed or finely chopped
1/3 cup almonds or cashews
1 cup fat-free half-and-half, or milk, or sour cream
Optional seasoning: 2 pinches nutmeg, or dash cinnamon, or 1/2–1 tsp each of thyme, marjoram, and basil, or 1 tsp sautéed ginger root
Optional garnish: Grated apple, toasted nuts, or yogurt

Directions

1. Peel and chop the carrots and place them in a medium-large saucepan with the stock, salt, and ginger paste. Bring to a boil, cover, and simmer until the vegetables are tender, about 12–15 minutes.

2. Heat butter in a small skillet. Add onions and sauté over medium heat for 5 minutes. Add garlic and optional seasoning herbs, and sauté about 5 minutes more, or until the onions are soft.

3. Purée everything together in a blender or food processor and transfer to a double boiler. Simmer gently 8–10 minutes. Whisk in dairy.

Illustration courtesy Paul McClendon, Age 12.

Nutrition information is with fat-free half-and-half and does not include optional ingredients.

Exchanges	Calories 122	Cholesterol 6 mg
3 Vegetable	Calories from Fat 44	Sodium 44p mg
1 Fat	Total Fat 5g	Total Carbohydrate 17 g
	Saturated Fat 1.4 g	Dietary Fiber 4 g
	Polyunsaturated Fat 0.8 g	Sugars 7 g
	Monounsaturated Fat 2.2 g	Protein 3 g

Yummy Chicken Tortellini Salad

Serving Size: about 1 cup
Total Servings: 8
Prep time: 20 minutes
Chill time: 2 hours or longer

Ingredients

3 1/2 cups combination of fresh or frozen chopped cauliflower, broccoli, carrots, red bell peppers, and water chestnuts—cooked according to package directions

1 package (9 oz) refrigerated uncooked cheese tortellini

3 cups cooked cubed chicken (leftovers work great)

1 (8 oz) bottle fat-free Italian dressing

2 Tbsp grated Parmesan cheese (freshly grated if possible)

> For a vegetarian version of this recipe, check out the Yummy Veggie Tortellini Salad on the next page!

Directions

1. If using fresh veggies, cook them in 2 Tbsp water in the microwave for about 3 minutes. Pierce with fork; if tender, they're done, If not, cook another 30 seconds and check again. (Water chestnuts are supposed to feel firm and taste crunchy when cooked, so test another vegetable.) Drain veggies and place in large bowl.

2. Cook tortellini according to package directions, then rinse in cold water, drain, and add to veggies in bowl. (Watch the tortellini carefully. If cooked too long, the filling starts seeping out.)

3. Add chicken and salad dressing to bowl, then combine all ingredients and toss gently to coat everything with dressing.

4. Cover bowl with lid, plastic wrap, or foil and refrigerate until chilled. Can be made the night before. Just before packing, sprinkle with cheese.

> **Timesaving Tip!**
> For convenience, you can substitute 3 cups canned chicken breast packed in water, drained, and separated into small chunks with a fork.

Exchanges	Calories 233	Cholesterol 60 mg
1 Starch	Calories from Fat 59	Sodium 492 mg
1 Vegetable	**Total Fat** 7 g	**Total Carbohydrate** 22 g
2 Lean Meat	Saturated Fat 2.4 g	Dietary Fiber 2 g
	Polyunsaturated Fat 1.4 g	Sugars 5 g
	Monounsaturated Fat 2.0 g	**Protein** 21 g

Yummy Veggie Tortellini Salad

 Serving Size: about 1 cup
Total Servings: 8
Prep time: 20 minutes
Chill time: 2 hours or longer

Ingredients

3 1/2 cups combination of fresh or frozen chopped cauliflower, broccoli, carrots, red bell peppers, and water chestnuts—cooked according to package Directions
1 package (9 oz) refrigerated uncooked cheese tortellini

Garlic Vinaigrette
1/3 cup cider or balsamic vinegar
1 Tbsp chopped fresh or 1 tsp dried basil leaves
3 Tbsp olive oil or vegetable oil
1/4 tsp paprika
1/8 tsp salt
1 clove garlic, finely chopped

1/2 cup grated carrots
2 cups broccoli florets

Directions

1. If using fresh veggies, cook them in 2 Tbsp water in the microwave for about 3 minutes. Pierce with fork; if tender, they're done, If not, cook another 30 seconds and check again. (Water chestnuts are supposed to feel firm and taste crunchy when cooked, so test another vegetable.) Drain veggies and place in large bowl.

2. Cook tortellini according to package directions, then rinse in cold water, drain, and add to veggies in bowl. (Watch the tortellini carefully. If cooked too long, the filling starts seeping out.)

3. Combine garlic vinaigrette ingredients in a jar with tight-fitting lid. Mix in carrots and broccoli florets.

4. Refrigerate pasta in a covered bowl and vinaigrette in jar overnight.

5. In the morning, combine veggies with vinaigrette. Gently mix in pasta.

Exchanges	Calories 177	Cholesterol 13 mg
1 Starch	Calories from Fat 70	Sodium 222 mg
1 Vegetable	Total Fat 8 g	Total Carbohydrate 22 g
1 1/2 Fat	Saturated Fat 2.0 g	Dietary Fiber 3 g
	Polyunsaturated Fat 1.0 g	Sugars 4 g
	Monounsaturated Fat 4.3 g	Protein 7 g

Fake 'n' Bake Pecan-Crusted Chicken

 Serving Size: 1
Total Servings: 4
Prep time: 20 minutes
Baking time: 40–50 minutes

Ingredients

2 Tbsp mustard (preferably Dijon)
2 Tbsp low-fat or regular Miracle Whip
1 Tbsp olive oil
1/2 tsp paprika
1/2 tsp Mrs. Dash or other herb seasoning
1 slice whole-wheat bread
1/2 cup chopped pecans or hazelnuts
1 Tbsp dried parsley flakes or 2 Tbsp chopped fresh parsley
4 skinless and boneless chicken breasts

Directions

1. Preheat oven to 375°F. Coat baking dish with nonstick cooking spray or oil.

2. Mix mustard, Miracle Whip, olive oil, paprika, and herb seasoning in medium bowl; set aside. Tear bread slice into chunks. Place bread, pecans, and parsley in food processor; pulse until mixture is finely ground.

3. Coat chicken with mustard mixture, then roll in crumb mixture; place in baking dish and bake for 40–50 minutes at 375°F.

Exchanges	Calories 339	Cholesterol 83 mg
1/2 Carbohydrate	Calories from Fat 180	**Sodium** 355 mg
4 Lean Meat	**Total Fat** 20 g	**Total Carbohydrate** 8 g
1 1/2 Fat	Saturated Fat 2.6 g	Dietary Fiber 2 g
	Polyunsaturated Fat 4.9 g	Sugars 2 g
	Monounsaturated Fat 10.9 g	**Protein** 33 g

Lentil Tortellini Salad

Serving Size: 1 cup
Total Servings: 7
Prep time: 45 minutes
Chilling time: 3 hours or more

Ingredients

Dressing
1/3 cup olive oil
1/3 cup balsamic vinegar or cider vinegar or other flavored vinegar
1/2 tsp salt
1/8 tsp black or white pepper
2 dashes hot pepper sauce or to taste
2 garlic cloves, minced

Salad
1 cup uncooked lentils
2 cups water
1 package (7 oz) uncooked plain tortellini
1/2 cup chopped fresh parsley
2 Tbsp chopped fresh oregano leaves or 2 tsp dried oregano leaves
1 medium tomato, seeded and chopped, or 4 sun-dried tomatoes packed in oil, wiped to remove oil
Optional: 1/2 cup thinly sliced green onions

Directions

1. Combine dressing ingredients in jar with tight-fitting lid and shake to blend well.

2. Sort and rinse lentils. Bring 2 cups water to boil in 2-quart saucepan; add lentils and reduce heat. Cover and simmer on low heat 15–20 minutes or until lentils are tender but not mushy. Drain.

3. While lentils cook, cook tortellini as directed on package. Drain and rinse with cold water. In large bowl, combine all salad ingredients and toss. Pour dressing over salad; toss again. Cover and refrigerate 3 hours or until chilled.

Protein Power

Adding chicken, turkey, or ham, or even small bits of salami, cooked sausage, or pepperoni would make this dish even more satisfying for a hungry teen. However, the combination of a legume (lentils) and a grain (tortellini) make this dish count as protein for kids who choose to eschew meat.

Exchanges	Calories 300	Cholesterol 0 mg
2 1/2 Starch	Calories from Fat 99	Sodium 173 mg
1 Very Lean Meat	**Total Fat** 11 g	**Total Carbohydrate** 41 g
1 1/2 Fat	Saturated Fat 1.5 g	Dietary Fiber 7 g
	Polyunsaturated Fat 1.2 g	Sugars 4 g
	Monounsaturated Fat 7.6 g	**Protein** 11 g

Fruit and Veggie
Side Dishes
and Snacks

Easy English Muffin Pizza

Serving Size: 2 muffin halves
Total Servings: 1
Prep time: 5 minutes
Baking time: 3–5 minutes

Ingredients
2 Tbsp pizza sauce or Italian tomato sauce
1 English muffin, split
2 Tbsp veggies of your choice (onions, broccoli, zucchini, mushrooms, garlic, or bell peppers)
2 Tbsp reduced-fat grated mozzarella cheese

Directions
1. Spread 1 Tbsp sauce on each English muffin half.
2. Cover muffins with veggies. Sprinkle grated cheese on top.
3. Broil pizzas 3–5 minutes or until the cheese melts. Heat about 1 minute in the microwave.

Groaner
Do you know why bakers' kids are so bored? They have muffin to do.

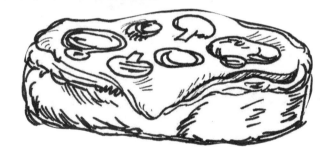

Exchanges	Calories 187	Cholesterol 7 mg
2 Starch	Calories from Fat 31	Sodium 488 mg
1/2 Fat	Total Fat 3 g	Total Carbohydrate 30 g
	Saturated Fat 1.4 g	Dietary Fiber 2 g
	Polyunsaturated Fat 0.9 g	Sugars 4 g
	Monounsaturated Fat 0.6 g	Protein 9 g

Fruit Leather

Serving Size: 1/6 of scroll
Total Servings: 6
Prep time: 30 minutes
Baking time: 4–5 hours
Drying time: 4–5 days

Ingredients
2 lb peaches, pears, apricots, or berries

Groaner
Did you see the movie *Wild Peaches*? It was rated peachy 13, and boy was it the pits.

Directions
1. Wash and pit or seed fruit. In a medium bowl, mash into a purée or use a blender.

2. Spread purée on cookie sheets evenly at 1-inch thickness and bake at 150°F for 4–5 hours. Dry until purée is firm and edges can be lifted easily.

3. Peel from cookie sheets while still warm and roll into scrolls.

4. Dry in paper or cloth bags for 4–5 days and then wrap in wax paper and store in airtight containers.

Exchanges	Calories 60	Cholesterol 0 mg
1 Fruit	Calories from Fat 4	Sodium 1 mg
	Total Fat 0 g	**Total Carbohydrate** 15 g
	Saturated Fat 0 g	Dietary Fiber 3 g
	Polyunsaturated Fat 0 g	Sugars 11 g
	Monounsaturated Fat 0 g	**Protein** 1 g

Eskimo Ice Cream

Serving size: 1/2 cup
Total Servings: 2
Prep time: 10 minutes
Chill time: 2 hours or more

Ingredients
1 cup any kind of berries, use frozen if eating immediately
1/2 cup nonfat plain or vanilla-flavored yogurt
pinch of fructose (other sweeteners may be substituted, if desired)
2 drops lemon juice, if desired

Directions
Blend all ingredients with a wire whisk, pulse in a food processor, or mix in blender for a smoother consistency. Freeze if made with fresh berries.

For a Nondairy Treat
Replace the nonfat yogurt with either rice or soy yogurt. Then we can all scream for ice cream!

Two Scoops of Caribou, Please
Long ago, Eskimos made their version of ice cream from berries mixed with animal oil from whales, seals, or walruses and frozen, grated dried fat from caribou, reindeer, or moose. They might add snow, fish, and greens, too. The Sioux Indians made a version with chokecherries and tallow. At one point in history, hydrogenated fat replaced the fauna scrapings. We've suggested other substitutions. As you can imagine, packing this one in a lunchbox could get pretty tricky, but for a summer vacation midday treat, it's perfect.

Exchanges	Calories 62	Cholesterol 1 mg
1/2 Fruit	Calories from Fat 4	Sodium 50 mg
1/2 Fat-Free Milk	Total Fat 0 g	Total Carbohydrate 12 g
	Saturated Fat 0 g	Dietary Fiber 4 g
	Polyunsaturated Fat 0 g	Sugars 6 g
	Monounsaturated Fat 0 g	Protein 4 g

Lime Mint Melon Salad

Serving Size: 1/2 cup
Total Servings: 6
Prep time: 20 minutes
Chill time: 2 hours or more

Ingredients
1 tsp honey or agave nectar
1 tsp lime juice
1 1/2 cups 1/2-inch cubes honeydew melon
1 1/2 cups 1/2-inch cubes cantaloupe
1 tsp grated lime peel
3 Tbsp very finely chopped fresh, or 1 Tbsp dried mint leaves

Directions
1. In a small bowl, blend honey or agave nectar with lime juice.

2. Toss all ingredients in medium glass or plastic bowl.

3. Cover and refrigerate about 2 hours or until chilled.

Melon Quiz
What do you call two melon sweethearts who can't marry?

CAN'T-ELOPE.

Exchanges
1/2 Fruit

Calories 34
  Calories from Fat 2
Total Fat 0 g
  Saturated Fat 0 g
  Polyunsaturated Fat 0 g
  Monounsaturated Fat 0 g

Cholesterol 0 mg
Sodium 12 mg
Total Carbohydrate 8 g
  Dietary Fiber 1 g
  Sugars 7 g
Protein 1 g

Lunchbox Banana Split

Serving Size: 1 banana split
Total Servings: 1
Prep time: 5 minutes

Ingredients

1 small banana
1 1/2 tsp peanut butter or other nut butter, if desired
1 Tbsp total from any of the following "sprinkles": sunflower seeds, granola, chopped nuts, coconut, raisins, raspberries, strawberries, dried cranberries, or coconut

Directions

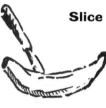

Slice

1. Slit the banana lengthwise down the middle, taking care not to cut all the way through the banana.

2. Spread the peanut butter on one half of the split side of the banana. Add the sprinkles, close the banana, tightly wrap the peel around the banana, and then trim both ends a bit to make it easier to peel at lunchtime. Banana shouldn't turn brown.

Fill

This great lunch idea was invented by lunch-packing dad, German Perico.

Peel & eat

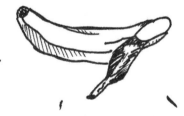

Nutrition information assumes sprinkles are equal parts sunflower seeds, granola, and chopped almonds.

Exchanges	Calories 168	Cholesterol 0 mg
2 Fruit	Calories from Fat 58	Sodium 47 mg
1 Fat	Total Fat 6 g	Total Carbohydrate 27 g
	Saturated Fat 1.3 g	Dietary Fiber 3 g
	Polyunsaturated Fat 2.3 g	Sugars 17 g
	Monounsaturated Fat 2.4 g	Protein 4 g

Peach & Peanut Butter Dipping Sauce

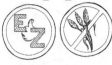

Serving Size: 1 1/2 tsp
Total Servings: 4
Prep time: 5 minutes

Ingredients
2 1/2 Tbsp natural peanut butter
4 Tbsp low-fat peach-flavored yogurt

Avoiding Culture Shock

Live yogurt cultures are nutritional dynamos. So how do you get them into that picky eater's diet? Serve them this dip with sticks of celery & jicama or a crispy apple. It's so easy, they can make it themselves.

Directions
1. Place the peanut butter in a microwave-safe container and zap it for about 30 seconds, just enough so it is easily stirred.

2. Add the yogurt and stir well.

3. Place in a container with a tight-fitting lid.

Exchanges	Calories 71	Sodium 46 mg
1/2 Carbohydrate	Calories from Fat 45	**Total Carbohydrate** 3 g
1 Fat	**Total Fat** 5 g	Dietary Fiber 1 g
	Saturated Fat 0.9 g	Sugars 1 g
	Polyunsaturated Fat 1.4 g	**Protein** 3 g
	Monounsaturated Fat 2.4 g	
	Cholesterol 0 mg	

Recipe is adapted from a recipe contributed by Lauri Ann Randolph, the award-winning author of Lauri's Low Carb Cookbook *and* Low Carb Creations from Lauri's Kitchen.

Celery Stuffing

Serving Size: 3 Tbsp stuffing and 4 celery sticks
Total Servings: 6
Prep time: 10 minutes

Ingredients
4 Tbsp grated carrot
4 Tbsp currants
2 tsp curry
1/2 cup cottage cheese
Optional: 2 Tbsp minced red pepper
24 5-inch celery sticks

Directions
1. Combine all ingredients except celery sticks with wooden spoon; stir until smooth.

2. Stuff celery sticks with mixture. Stuffing keeps for about a week.

Try It and Like It
We'll be the first to admit that this one can seem like a hard sell. But we happen to know a very picky teenage boy that devours these every time.

Exchanges	Calories 53	Cholesterol 3 mg
1/2 Carbohydrate	Calories from Fat 9	Sodium 130 mg
	Total Fat 1 g	Total Carbohydrate 8 g
	Saturated Fat 0.4 g	Dietary Fiber 2 g
	Polyunsaturated Fat 0.1 g	Sugars 6 g
	Monounsaturated Fat 0.3 g	Protein 3 g

Broccoli-Raisin Salad

Serving Size: 1/2 cup
Total Servings: 10
Prep Time: 15 minutes
Chilling Time: several hours

Ingredients

1 bunch broccoli (3 cups), rinsed, drained, and finely chopped
1 cup sunflower seeds (raw or unsalted dry roasted)
1 cup raisins
1/4 cup finely chopped red onion or chives
9 slices fried bacon, crumbled (can use low-salt version), or 1/4 cup bacon substitute

Dressing
1/2 cup nonfat mayonnaise
1 Tbsp apple cider vinegar
2 Tbsp fructose or sugar substitute

Directions

1. Place non-dressing ingredients in large bowl.

2. In medium bowl, mix dressing ingredients well.

3. Stir into salad ingredients and serve.

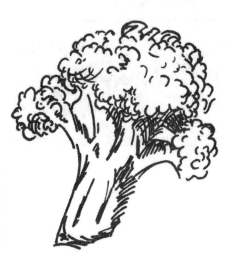

Time-Saving Tip

To save time, use packaged broccoli slaw and pulse in a food processor or a blender.

Exchanges	Calories 175	Cholesterol 6 mg
1 1/2	Calories from Fat 80	Sodium 224 mg
Carbohydrate	Total Fat 9 g	Total Carbohydrate 20 g
1 1/2 Fat	Saturated Fat 1.4 g	Dietary Fiber 3 g
	Polyunsaturated Fat 4.5 g	Sugars 14 g
	Monounsaturated Fat 2.3 g	Protein 6 g

Fruit Slaw

Serving Size: 2/3 cup
Total Servings: 6
Prep time: 15 minutes with a food processor, 15–20 minutes without

Ingredients

3 cups shredded cabbage
1 cup finely chopped apple
1/4 cup dried cranberries (substitute dried blueberries, if desired)
1 can (8 oz) crushed pineapple, well-drained, juice saved in small bowl or cup
1 cup plain nonfat yogurt
1 Tbsp honey

Yogurt Dressing
1/2 cup nonfat yogurt
2 Tbsp reserved pineapple juice
1 Tbsp honey
1 tsp Dijon mustard

Optional: unsalted, roasted, shelled sunflower seeds

Directions

1. Mix cabbage, apple, cranberries, and pineapple.

2. Mix ingredients for yogurt dressing. Stir in dressing, coating cabbage mixture well. If desired, sprinkle with sunflower seeds or pack them separately.

3. Mix all ingredients and chill until lunchtime. Can be made the night before.

Nutritional information does not include optional ingredients.

Exchanges	Calories 111	Cholesterol 1 mg
1 Fruit	Calories from Fat 4	Sodium 118 mg
1/2 Fat-Free Milk	Total Fat 0 g	Total Carbohydrate 24 g
	Saturated Fat 0 g	Dietary Fiber 2 g
	Polyunsaturated Fat 0 g	Sugars 20 g
	Monounsaturated Fat 0 g	Protein 4 g

Honey Peanut Slaw

Serving Size: 1/2 cup
Total Servings: 6
Prep time: 5 minutes
Chilling time: several hours

Ingredients

3 cups shredded cabbage
2 Tbsp finely chopped cilantro
1/3 cup small size peanuts or
  chopped large peanuts
1 Tbsp honey or fructose or sugar
  substitute
2 Tbsp rice vinegar
2 1/2 Tbsp canola oil
Optional: pinch red pepper flakes

Directions

1. Mix cabbage, cilantro, and peanuts in a large bowl.

2. Warm honey slightly in a small bowl in the microwave—about 15 seconds.

3. Mix honey and vinegar, then add to oil and stir to mix well. Pour over cabbage mix and stir gently to coat.

4. Chill up to several hours to blend flavors.

Appetizing Alternative!

For a creamy dressing, substitute
2 Tbsp nonfat plain yogurt
or low-fat mayonnaise for
the 2 Tbsp oil.

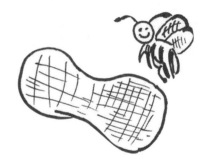

Illustration courtesy Anna McClendon, Age 10.

Exchanges	Calories 119	Cholesterol 0 mg
1/2 Carbohydrate	Calories from Fat 88	Sodium 73 mg
2 Fat	**Total Fat** 10 g	**Total Carbohydrate** 7 g
	Saturated Fat 1.3 g	Dietary Fiber 1 g
	Polyunsaturated Fat 3.0 g	Sugars 4 g
	Monounsaturated Fat 5.4 g	**Protein** 2 g

Kidney Bean Coleslaw

Serving Size: 1/2 cup
Total Servings: 8
Prep time: 10 minutes

Ingredients

3 cups shredded cabbage
1 can (8 oz) kidney beans, drained and rinsed
1/4 cup dill pickle relish or 1/4 cup sweet pickle relish
1/4 cup sliced green onions (optional)
1/4 cup non-fat mayonnaise or Miracle Whip
3 Tbsp mild salsa

Directions

1. Combine cabbage, kidney beans, relish, and onions.

2. Blend mayonnaise and salsa. Toss with cabbage mixture. Chill until lunchtime.

Exchanges	Calories 39	Cholesterol 0 mg
1/2 Carbohydrate	Calories from Fat 2	Sodium 195 mg
	Total Fat 0 g	Total Carbohydrate 7 g
	Saturated Fat 0 g	Dietary Fiber 2 g
	Polyunsaturated Fat 0 g	Sugars 2 g
	Monounsaturated Fat 0 g	Protein 2 g

Wake-Up-to-Breakfast Bean Dip

Serving size: 1/4 cup
Total Servings: 27
Prep time: 10 minutes
Cook time: 2 hours, or overnight

Ingredients

1 can (16 oz) nonfat refried beans
1 cup salsa
1 3/4 cup shredded reduced-fat cheddar cheese
3/4 cup plain nonfat yogurt
1 package (8 oz) nonfat cream cheese
2–3 tsp chili powder
1/4 tsp ground cumin

Directions

1. In slow cooker, mix the above ingredients.

2. Cover and cook on low overnight with 1/2 cup water on the bottom of the crock pot (this may not be necessary on newer models) or on high for about 2 hours. Stir once or twice.

Serving Tip

This recipe packs nicely in a thermos with baggies of chips or veggies of your choice and a little side of salsa.

Exchanges	Calories 48	Cholesterol 6 mg
1/2 Carbohydrate	Calories from Fat 15	**Sodium** 205 mg
1/2 Fat	**Total Fat** 2 g	**Total Carbohydrate** 4 g
	Saturated Fat 0.9 g	Dietary Fiber 1 g
	Polyunsaturated Fat 0.1 g	Sugars 1 g
	Monounsaturated Fat 0.5 g	**Protein** 4 g

"Let's Party!" Mix

Serving Size: 1/2 cup
Total Servings: 18
Prep time: 20 minutes
Baking time: 1 hour
Cooling time: 1 hour

Ingredients

1/4 cup corn oil spread, tub
1 clove pressed or minced garlic, or 1 tsp garlic powder
1/2 tsp seasoned salt
4 tsp Worcestershire sauce, or wheat-free tamari or soy sauce (San-J makes a version of this and has a reduced-sodium variety also)
3 cups rice squares cereal
3 cups corn squares cereal
3 cups wheat squares cereal, or Cheerios
1/2 cups raw almonds
1 cup pretzels
Optional: 1/2 cup bagel chips, small cheese crackers, or other small whole grain crackers

For Gluten-Free Shindigs

This can easily be made gluten-free with wheat-free tamari and gluten-free cereals.

Directions

1. Preheat oven to 250°F. In open roasting pan, melt margarine with pressed garlic in oven. Remove. Stir in seasoned salt and Worcestershire or soy sauce. Gradually add cereals, nuts, and pretzels, stirring until all pieces are evenly coated. (If you're using Cheerios, be sure they don't absorb too much butter, as they will shrink up and become, in cooking terms, yucky).

2. Bake 1 hour, stirring every 15 minutes. Cool about 1 hour. Store in airtight container.

This One's a Keeper

This tasty mix will freeze nicely for up to four months. Marie's grandma, Minnie, doubled this recipe and froze it in cereal boxes for when the grandkids dropped in.

Exchanges	Calories 99	Cholesterol 0 mg
1 Starch	Calories from Fat 39	Sodium 235 mg
1/2 Fat	Total Fat 4 g	Total Carbohydrate 14 g
	Saturated Fat 0.7 g	Dietary Fiber 1 g
	Polyunsaturated Fat 1.1 g	Sugars 1 g
	Monounsaturated Fat 2.2 g	Protein 2 g

Polenta with Bell Pepper Strips

Serving Size: 1/2 cup polenta, plus unlimited veggies
Total Servings: 8
Prep time: 20 minutes

Ingredients
2 1/4 cups cold water
1 cup tomato polenta mix (Fantastic brand works well)
7 Tbsp parmesan cheese, freshly shredded (cheddar cheese is good, too)
1 can (8 oz) of corn, drained
2 medium red bell peppers
2 medium orange bell peppers

Yummy Utensils
The curved ends of bell peppers make them the perfect utensils for eating the polenta, which is a thick cornmeal mush from our Italian friends. Most school kids will love this recipe, particularly this version that has extra cheese.

Directions
1. In a deep saucepan over high heat, add the water and the polenta mix. Bring to a boil then reduce heat and simmer for 5 minutes. Stir occasionally. Remove from heat, stir in the cheese and the corn. Allow to cool for about 10 minutes. Meanwhile, remove the stems from the peppers and cut into strips.
2. Place the polenta in a plastic container and the strips of bell pepper in a baggie.

Exchanges	Calories 142	Cholesterol 6 mg
1 Starch	Calories from Fat 33	**Sodium** 262 mg
1 Vegetable	**Total Fat** 4 g	**Total Carbohydrate** 23 g
1/2 Fat	Saturated Fat 1.4 g	Dietary Fiber 3 g
	Polyunsaturated Fat 0.8 g	Sugars 5 g
	Monounsaturated Fat 1.1 g	**Protein** 6 g

Adapted from a recipe contributed by Lauri Ann Randolph, the award-winning author of Lauri's Low Carb Cookbook *and* Low Carb Creations from Lauri's Kitchen.

Zesty Corn Dip

Serving size: 1/4 cup
Total Servings: 16
Prep time: 12 minutes

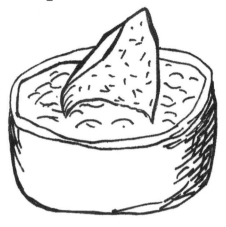

Ingredients

1 package (8 oz) fat-free cream
  cheese, softened
2 Tbsp lime juice
1 tsp ground red chilies
1 tsp ground cumin
2 Tbsp canola or safflower oil
1/4 tsp salt
dash of pepper, or 2 tsp mild salsa
1/2 cup whole kernel corn, drained
1/2 cup finely chopped walnuts or
  pecans
2 Tbsp onion, chopped (1/2 small
  onion)

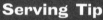

Directions

1. Using a beater, beat cream cheese,
   lime juice, chilies, cumin, oil, salt
   and pepper in large bowl on medium
   speed until smooth.

2. Stir in corn, walnuts, and onion.
   Serve with tortilla chips if desired.

Serving Tip

Celery or bell pepper slices make
nice scoopers. This is also great with
rice cakes, corn thins, pita bread,
or whole-grain crackers.

Exchanges	Calories 58	Cholesterol 2 mg
1 Fat	Calories from Fat 38	Sodium 123 mg
	Total Fat 4 g	Total Carbohydrate 3 g
	Saturated Fat 0.4 g	Dietary Fiber 0 g
	Polyunsaturated Fat 2.3 g	Sugars 1 g
	Monounsaturated Fat 1.4 g	Protein 3 g

Snacks
and Desserts

Fit for a King
Applesauce Spice Cake

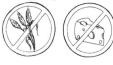

Serving Size: 3 x 4-inch piece
Total Servings: 12
Prep time: 15 minutes

Ingredients
3 cups barley flour
2 tsp baking soda
1 tsp salt
2 tsp cinnamon
1/2 tsp cloves
2 cups unsweetened applesauce (or other puréed fruit)
1/2 cup canola oil
1/2 cup honey
2 tsp vanilla

Directions
1. Sift together in medium bowl 3 cups barley flour, 2 tsp baking soda, 1 tsp salt, 2 tsp cinnamon, 1/2 tsp cloves.

2. In another bowl, mix together 2 cups applesauce (or other puréed fruit), 1/2 cup oil, 1/2 cup honey, and 2 tsp vanilla.

3. In large bowl, mix liquid with dry ingredients.

4. Bake in greased 9 x 13-inch pan in 350°F oven for 35–40 minutes, or 1 12-cup cupcake pan for 15–20 minutes, until a toothpick stuck into middle of cake comes out clean.

5. Let cool 10 minutes, remove from pan, and place on cake rack to cool.

Let Them (All) Eat Cake
For a gluten-free version of this recipe, replace the barley flour with gluten-free baking mix and omit the soda and the salt. This recipe comes straight from Woodrose Kindergarten in the Denver Waldorf School. This is their birthday cake standard, since it's a recipe most children can eat.

Exchanges	Calories 274	Cholesterol 0 mg
3 Carbohydrate	Calories from Fat 90	Sodium 407 mg
1 1/2 Fat	**Total Fat** 10 g	**Total Carbohydrate** 44 g
	Saturated Fat 0.8 g	Dietary Fiber 4 g
	Polyunsaturated Fat 3.1 g	Sugars 16 g
	Monounsaturated Fat 5.7 g	**Protein** 4 g

Not a Nutter Butter (But Close)

Serving Size: 1 sandwich cookie, **Total Servings:** 33
Prep time: 30 minutes
Baking time: 9–14 minutes per sheet
Cooling time: 20 minutes

Ingredients

2 1/2 cups flour (part or all whole grain flour)
1 tsp baking powder
1/4 tsp salt
1/2 cup corn oil spread, tub
1/3 cup unsweetened applesauce or 1 jar (4 oz) prune baby food
1/2 cup fructose
1/4 cup low-fat (1%) milk
1 egg
1 1/2 tsp vanilla or almond extract
1 1/4 cup rolled or 1 cup quick-cooking oats (organic tastes better!)

Filling
3/4 cup 100% peanut butter
1/2 cup 100% strawberry jam or grape jelly

Directions

1. Preheat oven to 375°F. Sift flour, baking powder, and salt into a large bowl.

2. Add margarine, applesauce or prunes, fructose, milk, egg, and extract. Beat with an electric mixer or with a wooden spoon until well-blended, 2–4 minutes. Gradually stir in rolled oats by hand unless you have a powerful mixer.

3. Roll out dough with rolling pin to 1/4-inch thickness. Cut out with a variety of cookie cutter shapes (be sure there's at least two of each shape to match for cookie sandwiches) and place on cookie baking sheets. Bake for about 9–14 minutes or until cookie springs back when touched. Do not over bake. Remove immediately and place on clean dry countertop lined with waxed paper or on wire racks. Cool 20 minutes.

4. Spread 1 generous tsp peanut butter and 1 not-so-generous tsp jam (so the jam doesn't drip) between 2 identical cookies.

Appetizing Alternative

Spread softened nonfat cream cheese instead of peanut butter for a creamy variation of this recipe.

Exchanges	Calories 132	Cholesterol 7 mg
1 Carbohydrate	Calories from Fat 55	Sodium 84 mg
1 Fat	**Total Fat** 6 g	Total Carbohydrate 17 g
	Saturated Fat 1.2 g	Dietary Fiber 2 g
	Polyunsaturated Fat 1.8 g	Sugars 6 g
	Monounsaturated Fat 2.8 g	**Protein** 4 g

Great Anytime Sweet Potato Knots

Serving Size: 1 knot
Total Servings: 12
Prep time: 2–2 1/2 hours
Baking time: 14–20 minutes

Ingredients

2 1/8 to 2 1/2 cups bread flour
 (may substitute 1/4 cup
 whole grain flour)
3 Tbsp fructose
1 tsp salt
1/2 tsp cinnamon
1 package quick active dry yeast
1/4 cup corn oil spread, tub
3/4 cup lukewarm water (95°F)
3/4 cup mashed, cooked, fresh sweet
 potatoes, drained if boiled
1/2 cup dried cranberries
1 Tbsp toasted wheat germ
1 Tbsp stick corn oil margarine, melted

Directions

1. In a large bowl, mix 1 cup of the flour,
 the fructose, salt, cinnamon, and yeast.
 Add 1/4 cup margarine and the warm
 water. Beat with electric mixer on low
 speed 1 minute, scraping bowl frequently. Add sweet potatoes. Beat on
 medium speed 1 minute, scraping bowl
 frequently. Stir in cranberries, wheat
 germ, and remaining flour, 1/4 cup at
 a time, until dough is easy to handle
 and doesn't stick to the fingers.

2. Place dough on lightly floured surface. Knead about 5 minutes, or until
 smooth and springy.
 Place dough in large
 bowl sprayed with veg-
 etable cooking spray or
 greased with oil, turn-
 ing dough to grease all
 sides. Cover and let
 rise in warm place 1
 hour to 1 hour 30 min-
 utes, or until double
 original size.

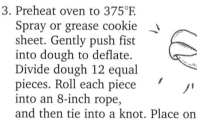

3. Preheat oven to 375°F.
 Spray or grease cookie
 sheet. Gently push fist
 into dough to deflate.
 Divide dough 12 equal
 pieces. Roll each piece
 into an 8-inch rope,
 and then tie into a knot. Place on
 cookie sheet.

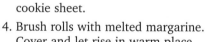

4. Brush rolls with melted margarine.
 Cover and let rise in warm place
 about 40 minutes or until double.
 Bake 14–20 minutes or until golden
 brown.

Timesaving Tip!

You may substitute canned, drained
mashed sweet potatoes for the fresh.

Exchanges
2 Starch
1/2 Fat

Calories 180
 Calories from Fat 47
Total Fat 5 g
 Saturated Fat 0.9 g
 Polyunsaturated Fat 1.7 g
 Monounsaturated Fat 2.2 g

Cholesterol 0 mg
Sodium 245 mg
Total Carbohydrate 30 g
 Dietary Fiber 2 g
 Sugars 8 g
Protein 3 g

Banana Nut Bread

Serving Size: 1 slice (1/2-inch)
Total Servings: 16
Prep time: 20 minutes
Baking time: 50–60 minutes

Ingredients
3 cups all-purpose flour (or 4 cups flour and no oat bran or wheat flour)
1/2 cup oat bran or whole grain flour
5 Tbsp granulated fructose or sugar substitute
2 tsp baking soda
2 eggs, beaten, or 1/2 cup egg substitute
4 large or 6 small ripe bananas, mashed (if not ripe enough, soften in microwave)
1/2 cup canola or safflower oil
2 tsp vanilla extract, or 1 tsp vanilla and 1 tsp almond extract
1 cup coarsely chopped walnuts
Optional: 1 Tbsp grated orange zest

Directions
1. Preheat oven to 350°F. Lightly grease 2 9 x 5-inch loaf pans.

2. In a medium bowl, whisk or sift together the flour, oat bran, fructose, and baking soda. Set aside. In a large bowl, beat together egg, bananas, oil, and vanilla. The mixing can be done by hand or with an electric mixer on slow to medium speed. Add the dry ingredients and beat thoroughly. Stir in walnuts and optional orange zest by hand.

3. The batter will be thick, so be sure to spread it evenly in the pan. Bake for 50–60 minutes, or until knife inserted in center comes out clean. If needed, bake a little longer, but do not over-bake or the bread will dry out.

This One's a Keeper
Banana Nut Bread keeps well. Freeze the whole loaf or, if you're usually in a hurry, freeze slices for quick morning preparation.

Exchanges	Calories 263	Cholesterol 26 mg
2 Carbohydrate	Calories from Fat 118	Sodium 167 mg
2 1/2 Fat	Total Fat 13 g	Total Carbohydrate 32 g
	Saturated Fat 1.3 g	Dietary Fiber 2 g
	Polyunsaturated Fat 5.9 g	Sugars 10 g
	Monounsaturated Fat 5.2 g	Protein 5 g

Recipe courtesy of Jean Wade, author of How Sweet It Is…Without the Sugar.

Breakfast Cookies

Serving Size: 1 cookie
Total Servings: 32
Prep time: 20 minutes
Baking time: 9–12 minutes per sheet of cookies

Ingredients

1/2 cup corn oil spread, tub
2/3 cup fructose
1 Tbsp molasses
1 cup crushed pineapple
1 jar (4 oz) prune baby food, or
1/2 cup applesauce
2 tsp vanilla
1 tsp maple flavoring (we like Mapleine)
1 cup all-purpose flour
1 cup whole-grain flour (whole-wheat pastry flour perhaps)
3/4 cup nonfat dry milk, whey, or soy powder
1 1/2 tsp cinnamon
1 tsp baking soda
2 cups oatmeal
1 cup dried currents
1 cup chopped walnuts, almonds, or pecans

Directions

1. Preheat oven to 350°F. Cream margarine, sugar, and molasses in a large bowl for 2 minutes.

2. Add crushed pineapple, prunes, vanilla, and maple flavoring and mix.

3. Add flour, dry milk, cinnamon, and baking soda and blend for 2 minutes.

4. Stir in oats, currents, and nuts.

5. Drop cookies onto a lightly oiled baking sheet using 1 Tbsp of dough for each cookie, and flatten slightly. Bake at 350°F for 9–12 minutes.

Tasty Tip!

This delicious cookie is an easy way to get oatmeal in kids at breakfast or any time. Some kids, though, don't care for the consistency of the pineapple. If so, blend the fruit in the blender for a smoother texture.

Exchanges	Calories 143	Cholesterol 0 mg
1 1/2 Carbohydrate	Calories from Fat 52	Sodium 79 mg
1 Fat	**Total Fat** 6 g	**Total Carbohydrate** 21 g
	Saturated Fat 0.8 g	Dietary Fiber 2 g
	Polyunsaturated Fat 2.8 g	Sugars 10 g
	Monounsaturated Fat 1.8 g	**Protein** 3 g

Chocolate Chip Cookies

Serving size: 1 cookie
Total Servings: 40
Prep time: 20 minutes
Baking time: 30–40 minutes

Ingredients

2 1/4 cups all-purpose flour
2 Tbsp toasted wheat germ or oat bran
1 tsp baking soda
1/2 cup corn oil spread, tub
3/4 cup fructose
1 Tbsp molasses
1 large egg
2 tsp real vanilla extract
1/2 cup mini chocolate chips
optional: 1/2 cup chopped walnuts, or one whole nut placed on top before baking

Directions

1. Preheat oven to 300°F. In medium bowl sift or combine flour, wheat germ, and soda.
2. In large bowl with electric mixer, beat margarine, molasses, and sugar very well. (Psst: The secret to great desserts is to really mix the fat and sugar together.)
3. Add egg and vanilla and beat well.
4. Mix in the flour mixture, then the chocolate chips, blending on low speed.
5. Drop by teaspoonfuls onto ungreased cookie sheets, 1 inch apart (20 cookies per sheet, cherry size balls). Try flattening the tops of cookies for a smooth look. Bake for 15–18 minutes until lightly browned. Immediately put cookies on a cooling rack.

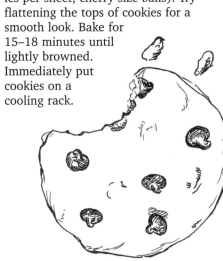

Tasty Tip!

The secret to moist low-fat cookies and cakes is to almost underbake them, cool, and store right away.

Appetizing Alternative

To drop the chocolate overload, we reduced the amount of chips and used mini chips instead. But if you're looking for a tasty way to drop the chocolate altogether, delete the chips and dip and press tops of dough in toffee (butter brittle) pieces.

Nutritional information does not include optional ingredients.

Exchanges	Calories 75	Cholesterol 5 mg
1 Carbohydrate	Calories from Fat 28	Sodium 57 mg
	Total Fat 3 g	Total Carbohydrate 11 g
	Saturated Fat 0.9 g	Dietary Fiber 0 g
	Polyunsaturated Fat 0.8 g	Sugars 5 g
	Monounsaturated Fat 1.3 g	Protein 1 g

Fry Bread

Serving Size: 1 fry bread
Total Servings: 10
Prep time: 15 minutes
Cooking time: 3–4 minutes

Ingredients

2 cups whole-wheat flour
2 cups white flour
4 level Tbsp baking powder
1 tsp salt
1/4 cup canola or safflower oil
1 cup warm water

Now That's Fusion

You can use this fry bread recipe to make a great Indian Taco. Simply put beans, shredded lettuce, tomato, and cheese (or non-dairy cheese) on top of fry bread and fold. The best of two cultures!

Directions

1. Mix together whole-wheat flour, white flour, baking powder, and salt. Add canola oil a little at a time, only enough to make the mixture look like corn meal.

2. Slowly add 1 cup warm water, only adding enough to make dough stick together. Roll into 10 fist-sized balls.

3. Cover the bowl with a towel for about 10 minutes. Pat dough out with your hands to the size of large pancakes.

4. Fry in hot oil until golden brown on both sides (about 375°F). Drain on paper towels.

Exchanges	Calories 265	Cholesterol 0 mg
2 1/2 Starch	Calories from Fat 97	Sodium 670 mg
1 1/2 Fat	Total Fat 11 g	Total Carbohydrate 38 g
	Saturated Fat 1.5 g	Dietary Fiber 4 g
	Polyunsaturated Fat 4.6 g	Sugars 1 g
	Monounsaturated Fat 4.5 g	Protein 6 g

This recipe graciously made available by the Nutrition and Dietetics Training Program of the Indian Health Service (IHS) in New Mexico.

Corny Cornbread

Serving Size: 1 slice
Total Servings: 12
Prep time: 15 minutes
Baking time: 20 minutes

Ingredients
1 1/2 cups yellow cornmeal
1/2 cup sifted all-purpose flour
2 Tbsp oat bran
1/4 tsp salt or less
1/2 tsp baking soda
2 tsp baking powder
Optional: 1/2–1 tsp chili powder, or
  1/4 teaspoon cayenne
1 cup low-fat buttermilk
1 egg
1/4 cup safflower or canola oil
Optional: up to 1 cup frozen corn,
  thawed and drained, or 1 can (12
  oz) whole kernel corn, drained

Appetizing Alternatives!

Confetti Cornbread: Add up to 1 cup of a combination of shredded sharp reduced-fat cheddar, finely grated carrots, and zucchini.

Corn Muffins: Grease a 12-cup muffin pan and divide batter among the cups. Bake 15–20 minutes.

Directions
1. Preheat oven to 425°F and set the oven rack on the second from bottom position. Spray with cooking spray or oil on a 9-inch square or round pan. (For a crispier crust, use the old-fashioned cast-iron skillet with a metal fireproof handle.) Warm the baking pan in the oven for about 5 minutes.

2. Put cornmeal, flour, oat bran, salt, baking soda, baking powder, and optional spices into a sifter and sift into a medium bowl.

3. In a medium bowl, beat egg slightly; add the buttermilk and oil. Pour over dry ingredients and beat well with a wooden spoon for just 30 seconds. Gently stir in optional corn.

4. With oven mitts, remove the hot pan from the oven. Gently pour and scrape the batter into the pan and gently shake pan to level batter.

5. Place the pan in the oven and bake for 20 minutes or until a toothpick inserted in the middle comes out clean. Let the cornbread set for a few minutes; cut into wedges or squares.

Tasty Tip!
Can be sliced for sandwich bread. Good with avocado, turkey, and lettuce.

Nutrition information does not include optional ingredients.

Exchanges	Calories 142	Cholesterol 18 mg
1 Starch	Calories from Fat 51	Sodium 189 mg
1 Fat	**Total Fat** 6 g	**Total Carbohydrate** 19 g
	Saturated Fat 0.6 g	Dietary Fiber 2 g
	Polyunsaturated Fat 1.6 g	Sugars 1 g
	Monounsaturated Fat 3.1 g	**Protein** 3 g

Honey Bran Muffins

Serving Size: 1 muffin
Total Servings: 6
Prep time: 10 minutes
Baking time: 15–20 minutes

Ingredients

1/4 cup wheat bran
3 Tbsp boiling water
1/4 cup low-fat (1%) milk
2 Tbsp packed brown sugar
2 Tbsp canola oil
2 Tbsp honey
1/4 cup fat-free, cholesterol-free egg
   product, or 2 egg whites
2/3 cup all-purpose flour
1 1/2 tsp baking powder
1/4 tsp salt
Optional: pinch granulated sugar

Directions

1. Preheat oven to 400°F. Spray 6 medium muffin cups with cooking spray or line with paper baking cups. In small bowl, mix wheat bran and boiling water; set aside.

2. In medium bowl, beat milk, brown sugar, oil, honey and egg product with spoon until well-mixed. Stir in bran mixture, flour, baking powder, and salt just until flour is moistened.

3. Divide batter evenly among muffin cups. If desired, sprinkle with granulated sugar. Bake 15–20 minutes until golden brown or tops spring back when touched lightly in center. Immediately remove from pan to wire rack.

Exchanges	Calories 145	Cholesterol 1 mg
1 1/2 Carbohydrate	Calories from Fat 44	Sodium 214 mg
1 Fat	**Total Fat** 5 g	**Total Carbohydrate** 24 g
	Saturated Fat 0.4 g	Dietary Fiber 2 g
	Polyunsaturated Fat 1.5 g	Sugars 11 g
	Monounsaturated Fat 2.8 g	**Protein** 3 g

Super-Duper Muffins

Serving Size: 1 muffin
Total Servings: 12
Prep time: 15 minutes
Baking time: 20 minutes

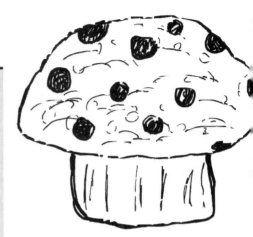

Ingredients
2 cups all-purpose flour
2/3 cup fructose
1 Tbsp baking powder
1/4 tsp salt
1/2 tsp cinnamon
1 1/2 cups finely chopped Granny Smith apples
Optional fruit/vegetable: dried blueberries, finely grated carrots and/or zucchini, rhubarb, finely chopped dried fruit
1/2 cup golden raisins or dried cranberries
2 eggs
1 cup low-fat buttermilk or low-fat (1%) milk
2 Tbsp corn oil spread, melted
1/2 tsp pure vanilla extract
Optional: pinch cinnamon-sugar mix

Directions
1. Place oven rack in top third of oven position. Preheat oven to 400°F. Spray 2-1/2–inch muffin pan with cooking spray, including top of pan.

2. Mix flour, fructose, baking powder, and salt with a wire whisk in a large bowl. Stir in the apple and raisins.

3. In medium bowl whisk eggs, milk, margarine, and vanilla until blended. Pour liquid mixture over dry and fold in with a spatula, just until combined.

4. Spoon batter into prepared cups. If desired, sprinkle cinnamon-sugar mix over muffin tops.

5. Bake 20 minutes. Turn out onto rack and serve warm or at room temperature.

Illustration courtesy Anna McClendon, Age 10.

Exchanges	Calories 212	Cholesterol 36 mg
2 1/2 Starch	Calories from Fat 46	Sodium 224 mg
1/2 Fat	**Total Fat** 5 g	**Total Carbohydrate** 38 g
	Saturated Fat 1.1 g	Dietary Fiber 2 g
	Polyunsaturated Fat 1.4 g	Sugars 19 g
	Monounsaturated Fat 2.1 g	**Protein** 4 g

Good Anytime Granola Bars

Serving Size: 1 bar
Total Servings: 48
Prep time: 15 minutes
Baking time: 25–30 minutes

Ingredients

3 cups old-fashioned or quick-cooking oats
1 cup finely chopped almonds
1/2 cup dried cranberries
1/2 cup finely chopped dried apricots
1 cup roasted, unsalted sunflower seeds
2 tsp cinnamon
7 Tbsp butter, melted
1 can (14 oz) fat-free sweetened condensed milk
1 tsp real vanilla extract

Directions

1. Preheat oven to 325°F. Line a 15 x 10-inch jelly roll pan with foil. Spray foil lightly with oil.

2. In large bowl, combine oats, almonds, cranberries, apricots, sunflower seeds, and cinnamon. In small bowl, combine butter, condensed milk, and vanilla. Pour over dry ingredients and mix well.

3. Press evenly into prepared jelly roll pan. Bake 25–30 minutes or until golden brown. Cool slightly; remove from pan and peel off foil. Cut into bars. Makes 48 bars.

Appetizing Alternatives!

This tasty treat is great for those who can't eat wheat and those who normally don't like oatmeal, too! To keep things interesting, try different combinations of nuts and dried fruits, such as tropical mix and macadamia nuts or cashews, pecans and cranberries or blueberries, or peanuts and golden raisins. If you want to boost the nutrition (and your lunchboxer can eat wheat), replace 1 Tbsp of the oats with 1 Tbsp toasted wheat germ or flaxseed meal.

Groaner

Where would the police put a health-nut crook?

Behind **granola** bars.

Exchanges	Calories 93	Cholesterol 4 mg
1 Carbohydrate	Calories from Fat 40	Sodium 21 mg
1/2 Fat	**Total Fat** 4 g	**Total Carbohydrate** 11 g
	Saturated Fat 1.4 g	Dietary Fiber 1 g
	Polyunsaturated Fat 1.4 g	Sugars 7 g
	Monounsaturated Fat 1.7 g	**Protein** 3 g

Little Fruit Pies

Serving Size: 1 fruit pie
Total Servings: 36
Prep time: A leisurely afternoon (or 1 hour with help)
Baking time: 20 minutes each
Chilling time: 2 hours

Ingredients

Pastry

2 cups low-gluten pastry or all-purpose
  flour
1/2 tsp salt
2 tsp fructose
1/2 cup corn oil spread,
  room temperature
8 oz fat-free cream cheese, room
  temperature
Optional: 1–2 Tbsp ice water

Pumpkin Filling

1 can (1 lb) pumpkin (not pumpkin
  pie mix)
1/3 cup fructose mixed with 1 tsp
  molasses
1/4 cup toasted ground almonds, or
  1/4 cup chopped golden raisins
1 tsp ginger purée, or 1 Tbsp finely
  chopped candied ginger

1/2 tsp cinnamon
1 tsp vanilla

Apricot-Pineapple Filling

2 packages (6 oz each) dried
  apricots
1 cup water
1 can (8 oz) crushed pineapple with
  juice
1/2 cup 100% fruit apricot
  preserves
1/4–1/3 cup fructose
1/8 tsp salt
4–6 Tbsp plain dried bread crumbs
  mixed with 1 tsp toasted
  wheat germ

Glaze

1 egg
1 Tbsp water
4 tsp fructose

Directions

Pastry

1. In a food processor, pulse the flour,
   salt, and fructose for 10 seconds.
   Add margarine and cream cheese;
   pulse as little as possible to get the
   desired effect. Add water, a little at a
   time, only if the dough doesn't hold
   together. (You can also use a pastry
   blender or two table knives to cut the
   fat into the dry ingredients, but it's
   more tedious.) Pulse until dough
   begins to clump together, but before
   it becomes a ball. Work dough as little as possible; divide dough into two
   balls, wrap in plastic and chill at
   least two hours or overnight.

2. Preheat oven to 375°F. Remove one
   dough ball to a floured surface and

   roll it out to about 1/8-inch thickness. Cut into rounds with a 3-inch
   cutter, flouring the cutter as
   needed.

Pumpkin Filling

Blend all ingredients in a medium
bowl.

Apricot-Pineapple Filling

1. In a heavy pan, place dried apricots,
   cover with water, and add the rest of
   the ingredients except bread crumbs.
   Simmer over medium heat until the
   apricots are very soft and liquid in
   pan.

2. Purée the mixture in a food processor
   or a blender (a little at a time) and
   add 4 Tbsp of bread crumbs and

combine. If filling isn't stiff, add more crumbs until it's firm but moist.

Glaze

1. To prepare glaze, whisk together the egg and water in a small bowl.

2. With a pastry brush, paint a light coat of glaze over each fruit pie and sprinkle them with fructose.

Pie

1. Place about 1 Tbsp filling near center of each prepared round. Fold pies in half, pinch edges to seal, and crimp (mash the edges together) with a fork. Place about 1 dozen pies on an ungreased, 12 x 15-inch cookie sheet. Repeat with other ball of dough, making sure to add more flour to rolling surface if necessary.

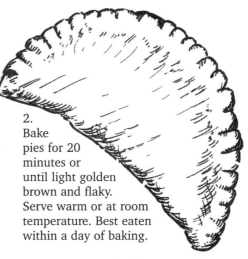

2. Bake pies for 20 minutes or until light golden brown and flaky. Serve warm or at room temperature. Best eaten within a day of baking.

Worth the Wait

This recipe can take a little while, but it's a much healthier substitute for those store-bought snack pies. Kids can cut out the circles, fill them, and seal the pies by mashing the edges together with fork tines. They're popular in Mexican and Native American cuisine.

With Pumpkin Filling

Exchanges	Calories 68	Cholesterol 7 mg
1/2 Starch	Calories from Fat 22	Sodium 85 mg
1/2 Fat	Total Fat 2 g	Total Carbohydrate 10 g
	Saturated Fat 0.4 g	Dietary Fiber 1 g
	Polyunsaturated Fat 1.0 g	Sugars 3 g
	Monounsaturated Fat 0.8 g	Protein 2 g

With Apricot-Pineapple Filling

Exchanges	Calories 94	Cholesterol 7 mg
1 Carbohydrate	Calories from Fat 25	Sodium 108 mg
1/2 Fat	Total Fat 3 g	Total Carbohydrate 16 g
	Saturated Fat 0.5 g7	Dietary Fiber 1 g
	Polyunsaturated Fat 0.8 g	Sugars 8 g
	Monounsaturated Fat 1.2 g	Protein 2 g

Fab Brownies

Serving Size: 1 square
Total Servings: 30
Prep time: 20 minutes
Baking time: 20–25 minutes

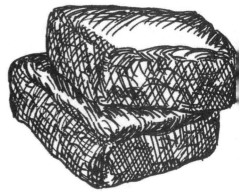

Ingredients
1 cup all-purpose flour
1/4 cup oat bran
5 Tbsp unsweetened cocoa
1 tsp baking powder
1/2 cup corn oil spread, tub
3/4 cup fructose
1 egg, beaten
1 tsp almond extract or flavoring
1 tsp vanilla extract
1 cup peeled, diced apple
  (1 medium)
optional: 1/2 cup chopped walnuts or
  pecans

Directions

1. Preheat oven to 350°F. Oil a 9 x 9-inch square pan. Sift or whisk together the flour, oat bran, cocoa, and baking powder very thoroughly.

2. In a large bowl, beat together spread and fructose. Add egg, almond extract, and vanilla extract. Pour the wet mixture into the dry ingredients. Mix thoroughly and then stir in chopped apple and nuts, if desired.

3. Spoon the brownie batter into the prepared pan. Bake brownies for 20–25 minutes or until brownies just pull away from sides. DO NOT OVERBAKE. Cool on rack and cut into 1-3/4–inch squares.

> This great recipe is the creation of Jacob McClendon, age 12.

Nutritional information does not include optional ingredients.

Exchanges	Calories 67	Cholesterol 8 mg
1/2 Carbohydrate	Calories from Fat 24	Sodium 37 mg
1/2 Fat	**Total Fat** 3 g	**Total Carbohydrate** 10 g
	Saturated Fat 0.6 g	Dietary Fiber 1 g
	Polyunsaturated Fat 1.2 g	Sugars 6 g
	Monounsaturated Fat 0.7 g	**Protein** 1 g

Shortbread Jam Cookies

Serving Size: 1 cookie
Total Servings: 32
Prep time: 25 minutes
Baking time: 10–20 minutes

Ingredients

1/2 cup corn oil spread, tub
3 Tbsp granulated fructose, or 2 tsp sugar substitute
1/2 tsp almond or vanilla extract
1 1/2 cups all-purpose flour or gluten-free baking mix
Optional: 1 Tbsp finely ground almonds
2 Tbsp no-sugar-added, raspberry, apricot, or blueberry jam

Directions

1. Preheat oven to 375°F. In a medium bowl, beat together margarine, fructose, and almond extract until soft, pale, and fluffy.

2. Gradually add flour in small amounts. Beat until smooth. When it becomes thick, knead with your hands until smooth. Knead in a bit more flour if it's too sticky, but it should be just right. Form a ball in the bowl.

3. From the dough ball, pull off pieces the size of a rounded teaspoon and place 1/2 inch apart on a large baking sheet. Form 32 dough balls. Do not flatten. After positioning all the balls, use your index finger to slightly indent each cookie and add a small dab of jam.

4. Bake 15–25 minutes, until edges are lightly golden. Do not overcook! Remove from oven. Cool 10 minutes. Transfer cookies to paper towels on rack. Store in airtight container lined with waxed paper, with waxed paper between layers, at room temperature.

Jean Wade's Most Popular Cookie!

The chefs for Holland America Line cruise ships used this recipe for a sugarless cookie choice. The chefs were surprised to find that even folks who could eat sugar went for the sugar-free varieties after tasting. The cookies made with sugar were almost untouched!

Exchanges	Calories 51	Cholesterol 0 mg
1/2 Carbohydrate	Calories from Fat 26	Sodium 0 mg
1/2 Fat	Total Fat 3 g	Total Carbohydrate 6 g
	Saturated Fat 0.5 g	Dietary Fiber 0 g
	Polyunsaturated Fat 0.9 g	Sugars 1 g
	Monounsaturated Fat 1.3 g	Protein 1 g

This recipe is courtesy of Jean Wade, author of How Sweet It Is…Without the Sugar. *(She vigorously beats all her ingredients by hand, a great way to add fun exercise, too.)*

Quick & Easy Pumpkin Pudding

Serving Size: 1/2 cup
Total Servings: 6
Prep time: 5 minutes
Microwaving time: 1 minute

Ingredients
8 oz fat-free cream cheese
1 can (15 oz) pumpkin (not pumpkin pie mix)
1/4 cup sugar substitute, or 3 Tbsp of honey or maple syrup
1/2 tsp pumpkin pie spice, or 1/4 tsp cinnamon and 1/4 tsp ginger

Directions
1. In a microwave-safe bowl, add the package of cream cheese (and the honey if using that) and zap for about 20 seconds, just enough so that the cream cheese is soft and easy to stir.
2. Add the pumpkin, sweetener and spices. Mix well.
3. Zap in the microwave again for about 30 seconds. Stir well. Taste test and add more sweetener or spices if desired.
4. Place in individual serving containers and refrigerate or freeze them until ready to add to a lunchbox.

Sneak Attack
Kids get a dessert that counts as a serving of vegetables (not that you need to tell them)! This pudding is rich in B vitamins, too.

Groaner
How do you mend a cracked jack-o-lantern?

With a pumpkin patch.

Exchanges	Calories 62	Cholesterol 4 mg
1/2 Carbohydrate	Calories from Fat 2	Sodium 205 mg
1 Very Lean Meat	**Total Fat** 0 g	**Total Carbohydrate** 9 g
	Saturated Fat 0 g	Dietary Fiber 2 g
	Polyunsaturated Fat 0 g	Sugars 4 g
	Monounsaturated Fat 0 g	**Protein** 6 g

Recipe is courtesy of Lauri Ann Randolph, the award-winning author of Lauri's Low Carb Cookbook *and* Low Carb Creations from Lauri's Kitchen.

Write-Your-Own-Fortune Cookies

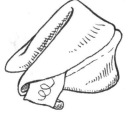

Serving Size: 1 cookie
Total Servings: 20
Prep time: 10 minutes
Baking time: 3 1/2–4 1/2 minutes

Ingredients

Butter or cooking spray for
  preparing pan
1/2 cup sifted all-purpose flour
1/2 cup fructose or sugar substitute
1/4 tsp salt
2 large egg whites at room
  temperature
1/2 tsp canola or safflower oil
1/2 tsp almond or vanilla extract
Optional: 1/4 tsp finely grated lemon
  or orange peel

Directions

1. Position rack in center of oven and preheat to 400°F. Spray or butter the cookie sheets.

2. Press the top of a 3-inch diameter glass upside down onto greased cookie sheets, making rings about 1 inch apart. It's best to have a ratio of 1 person helping per 2 hot cookies, as they will cool quickly and will no longer be pliable.

3. In large bowl of electric mixer, combine all ingredients and beat on medium speed just until batter is smooth; about 1-2 minutes.

4. Drop 1 tsp batter into center of each circle, using the back of a teaspoon dipped into cold water, spread the batter, filling but not overshooting the circle stamp.

5. Bake 3 1/2 to 4 1/2 minutes, watching them carefully and removing with oven mitts as soon as the edges are barely starting to brown. Set cookie sheet on a wire rack and immediately begin shaping one cookie at a time, using a spatula or pancake turner to slide the cookie off the sheet and turn the cookie upside down.

6. Place a paper fortune in center of cookie and fold in half over the paper. Grasp both ends of the cookie, place the middle of the folded edge on the rim of a bowl or measuring cup, and gently but firmly pull down on the ends to curve the top edge to make it fold if it doesn't happen to automatically while bending. Hold the curve for a few seconds, then set the cookie, tips down, into the cup of a muffin pan to cool and crisp completely. Let pans cool, clean, re-butter, and then repeat steps, using all the batter. Store in airtight container.

Exchanges	Calories 32		Cholesterol 0 mg
1/2 Carbohydrate	Calories from Fat 1		Sodium 35 mg
	Total Fat 0 g		Total Carbohydrate 7 g
	Saturated Fat 0 g		Dietary Fiber 0 g
	Polyunsaturated Fat 0 g		Sugars 5 g
	Monounsaturated Fat 0 g		Protein 1 g

Carrot or Zucchini Muffins

Serving Size: 1 muffin
Total Servings: 24
Prep time: 25 minutes
Baking time: 25 minutes

Ingredients

1/2 cup cold pressed or expeller pressed canola oil (ideal)
1/2 cup fructose, honey, pure maple syrup, or sugar substitute
2 eggs or 4 egg whites, beaten
1 tsp vanilla
1 1/2 cups grated zucchini, carrots, or both
2 1/2 tsp cinnamon, or to taste
1/2 tsp salt
1/2 cup flax meal (ground flaxseeds)
1 cup brown rice flour
1/3 cup buckwheat flour
1/2 tsp baking soda
1/2 tsp baking powder
1/2 cup chopped walnuts, almonds, or pecans

Directions

1. Preheat oven to 350°F. Line cupcake pans with paper cups.

2. Beat together oil and sweetener.

3. Add eggs, vanilla, and zucchini. Mix well.

4. Add dry ingredients. Stir in nuts.

5. Bake for about 25 minutes, until a toothpick stuck in the center comes out clean. Makes 2 dozen.

Tasty Tip!

These muffins freeze well. For ready-made muffins, double the batch and freeze half. If your family can eat gluten, substitute wheat flour for the flours listed above.

Exchanges	Calories 124	Cholesterol 18 mg
1 Carbohydrate	Calories from Fat 69	Sodium 95 mg
1 1/2 Fat	Total Fat 8 g	Total Carbohydrate 12 g
	Saturated Fat 0.7 g	Dietary Fiber 2 g
	Polyunsaturated Fat 3.2 g	Sugars 5 g
	Monounsaturated Fat 3.4 g	Protein 2 g

Adapted from certified nutritionist Karen Falbo's Vital Abundance Cooking Series.

Brown Rice Pudding

Serving Size: 1/2 cup
Total Servings: 11
Prep time: 15 minutes
Baking time: 45–60 minutes

Ingredients

1 1/2 cups nut milk (see Whole
Almond Milk recipe on page 130),
rice milk, or soy milk
2 eggs
1/2 cup agave nectar, or 1/3 cup
honey or maple syrup
1 tsp vanilla extract
1/2 tsp cinnamon
1/4 tsp allspice or nutmeg
Optional: 1/2 tsp cloves
1/2 cup raisins or dried currents
2 cups cooked brown rice or white
basmati rice
1/2 cup chopped almonds

Directions

1. Pre-heat oven to 350°F. Beat milk,
eggs, and sweetener together. Add
seasonings, raisins, and brown rice.

2. Pour into a greased 2-1/2–quart
casserole dish, sprinkle almonds on
top.

3. Bake for 45–60 minutes, until slightly
brown. Serve warm or cold.

All Inclusive

We didn't miss the dairy and we'll
bet you won't either (though, feel
free to slip it back in if it's not a
problem). This is great comfort food
you can enjoy without cheating.

Exchanges	Calories 188	Cholesterol 38 mg
1 1/2	Calories from Fat 73	Sodium 26 mg
Carbohydrate	Total Fat 8 g	Total Carbohydrate 25 g
1 1/2 Fat	Saturated Fat 0.9 g	Dietary Fiber 3 g
	Polyunsaturated Fat 1.8 g	Sugars 15 g
	Monounsaturated Fat 4.9 g	Protein 5 g

Recipe adapted with permission from Vital Abundance Cooking Series, *by Karen Falbo.*

Spicy Raisin Bean Muffins

 Serving Size: 1 muffin
Total Servings: 12
Prep time: 10 minutes
Baking time: 15–18 minutes

Ingredients
1 cup cooked pinto beans (canned beans, drained and rinsed, can be used)
3/4 cup low-fat (1%) milk
2 egg whites
1/4 cup canola oil (or 2 Tbsp oil and 2 Tbsp applesauce)
1/2 cup brown sugar (people with diabetes could substitute fructose and a bit of molasses)
1/2 tsp cinnamon
1/4 tsp nutmeg
1/4 tsp ground cloves
2 tsp baking powder
1/2 tsp baking soda
1 1/2 cup flour (part whole-wheat flour can be used)
1/2 cup raisins

Directions
1. Puree beans and milk in a blender until smooth.

2. Beat egg whites, oil, and brown sugar. Add bean mixture, spices, baking powder, and baking soda and mix well. Add flour and raisins and mix until just moistened.

3. Spoon into muffin cups. Bake at 400°F for 15–18 minutes or until golden.

Words of Wisdom

Diane Moyer, MS, RD, CDE, who specializes in the treatment of Celiac Disease in Denver, generously offered this recipe. When asked what she would like to have mentioned in a book such as this, she replied, *"I agree with the message promoting the low-fat diet. Unfortunately, it has gotten maligned by the current low-carb craze. I think the part of the message that got lost was the recommendation for complex carbohydrate foods— whole grains, fruits, and vegetables. Often people buy low-fat foods, but just get foods high in sugar and refined white flour, such as pasta, pretzels, bagels, and bars. I encourage people to choose an overall balanced diet, focusing more on produce, beans, and whole grains."*

Exchanges	Calories 181	Cholesterol 1 mg
2 Carbohydrate	Calories from Fat 46	Sodium 134 mg
1 Fat	**Total Fat** 5 g	**Total Carbohydrate** 30 g
	Saturated Fat 0.5 g	Dietary Fiber 2 g
	Polyunsaturated Fat 1.5 g	Sugars 14 g
	Monounsaturated Fat 2.9 g	**Protein** 4 g

Thumbs-Up Easy Chocolate Pound Cupcakes

Serving Size: 1 cupcake
Total Servings: 24
Prep time: 10 minutes
Bake time: 20 minutes

Ingredients
1 plain devil's food cake mix (18 1/4 oz) with no added pudding or oil
1 cup water
1/2 cup unsweetened applesauce
3/4 cup Egg Beaters or other egg substitute, or 5 egg whites
1–2 tsp cinnamon
Optional frosting: "Fat Free Naturally" Hot Fudge Sauce (we use Oh, Fudge! by Wax Orchard), peanut butter, or colorful sprinkles.

Your Call
You may use 3 whole eggs or a gluten-free cake mix if you want. The yolkless version rises a bit less and isn't quite as moist, but adults and children said they liked the chocolate taste better.

Directions
1. Place oven rack in middle position and preheat oven to 325°F. Place cupcake liners in a cupcake pan.

2. Place the cake mix, water, applesauce, cinnamon, and egg substitute in a large mixing bowl. Mix on low speed for 1 minute. Stop the mixer and scrape down the sides of the bowl. Beat 2 minutes on the middle speed. Spoon thick batter into the prepared cupcake pan. If using sprinkles, sprinkle on before baking.

3. Bake for 20 minutes. Cake is done if it springs back when lightly pressed with a fingertip. Cool for 10 minutes or so. Frost with optional low-fat hot fudge sauce or warm peanut butter.

Nutrition information does not include optional frosting.

Exchanges	Calories 93	Cholesterol 0 mg
1 Carbohydrate	Calories from Fat 22	Sodium 234 mg
1/2 Fat	Total Fat 2 g	Total Carbohydrate 17 g
	Saturated Fat 1.2 g	Dietary Fiber 1 g
	Polyunsaturated Fat 0.4 g	Sugars 9 g
	Monounsaturated Fat 0.8 g	Protein 2 g

Whole Almond Milk

Serving Size: 1/2 cup
Total Servings: 5
Prep time: 15 minutes
Soaking Time: 8–12 hours

Ingredients
1/2 cup dry almonds or less
4 cups water

Sweetening the Pot
If a sweeter milk is preferred, add 1 date to every 8 almonds plus 1 tsp vanilla.

Directions
1. Soak almonds in about 2 cups water in a medium bowl for 8–12 hours or overnight.

2. Drain and discard the water. Put just the almonds in a blender for 2 minutes on high. Add 2 cups of water and blend on high for another 2 minutes.

3. Optional: Pour through a cheese-cloth-lined strainer over the bowl for about 5 minutes. (Double-layer the cheesecloth.) Then fold the cheesecloth; and squeeze out the creamy rich fluid.

Nutrition information does not include optional straining.

Exchanges	Calories 82	Cholesterol 0 mg
1 1/2 Fat	Calories from Fat 66	Sodium 0 mg
	Total Fat 7 g	Total Carbohydrate 3 g
	Saturated Fat 0.6 g	Dietary Fiber 2 g
	Polyunsaturated Fat 1.7 g	Sugars 1 g
	Monounsaturated Fat 4.6 g	Protein 3 g

Recipe generously offered by Dawn Archer, a certified nutritionist.

Part Four:
More Food for Thought

Resources, Product Sources, and Websites

More Food for Thought

Resources, Product Sources, and Web Sites

Following are some resources, books, websites, and products we really like. There's obviously a lot more information out there than what we have listed here, but hopefully this will be a good start for health-conscious parents. Keep in mind that while these are sources we turn to for insight, we do not endorse nor ensure the validity of any of the products, advice, or information provided by these resources. Parents should use the information provided by these entities at their own discretion.

Bundles of Books

Children's storybooks for ages four through eight

The Berenstain Bears and Too Much Junk Food. Berenstain, Stan and Jan. Random House, 1985.
A well-known favorite found in most libraries.

D.W. the Picky Eater. Brown, Marc. Little, Brown & Company, 1995.
D.W. must overcome her distrust of new foods so she can go out to dinner to celebrate Grandma Thora's birthday. Can she do it?

I Will Never Not Ever Eat a Tomato. Child, Lauren. Candlewick Press, 2000.
Lola refuses to eat tomatoes. What will get her to try one?

Tawny Scrawny Lion. Jackson, Kathryn. Golden Books, 1997.
  Subtle vegetarian tale. The lion helps rabbits fill the pot of carrot stew. See our recipe for Tawny Scrawny Lion Soup on page 84.

No More Vegetables! Rubel, Nicole. Farrar, Straus and Giroux, 2002.
  This great little book illustrates how involving children with planting and gardening can promote healthy eating.

Gregory, the Terrible Eater. Sharmat, Mitchell. Simon & Schuster Children's Publishing, 1984.
  Mom and Dad goat get upset when their kid, Gregory, prefers nutritious food instead of tin cans. Nice twist on the usual parent-child food struggle.

Green Eggs and Ham. Dr. Seuss. Random House Books for Young Readers, 1960.
  Sam-I-Am chases a reluctant diner from the tops of trees to the bottom of the ocean to get him to try green eggs and ham in this wacky rhyming classic.

Eat Your Peas, Louise! Snow, Pegeen. Children's Press, 1985.
  After many attempted bribes fail to get Louise to eat her peas, her dad's best idea is just to say please. A short and sweet story about power struggles over food in a reading level for rookie readers.

Books for older children

Kids Cooking – A Very Slightly Messy Manual. Editors of Klutz. Klutz, 1987.

Pyramid Pal, et. al. Norton, Susan, and Dawson, Susan. Griffin Publishing Inc., 2000.
  A great series of books based on the nutrition recommendations of the USDA Food Guide Pyramid.

Books for parents

Little Sugar Addicts – End the Mood Swings, Meltdowns, Tantrums, and Low Self-Esteem in Your Child Today. DesMaisons, Kathleen, Ph.D. Three Rivers Press, 2004.
  The up-to-date info and thoroughness of this book are impressive.

Cookbooks

The New Enchanted Broccoli Forest. Revised Edition. Katzen, Mollie. Ten Speed Press, 2000.
  Tasty vegetarian soups included. Also has section for non-dairy, vegan, and "kid pleasers."

Beyond Macaroni and Cheese. Lagerborg, Mary Beth, and Parks, Karen. Zondervan Publishing Company, 1998.
Tasty, quick recipes to coax picky eaters. Tested by MOPS (Moms of Pre-Schoolers). Some recipes need healthier substitutions.

High Altitude Baking: 200 Delicious Recipes & Tips for Great Cookies, Cakes, Breads & More: For People Living Between 3,500 and 10,000 Feet. Kendall, Patricia, and the Colorado State University Cooperative Extension. 3D Press, 2003.
Nutritional Info for all the recipes in the back of the book.

101 Things to Do with Ramen Noodles. Patrick, Toni. Gibbs Smith, 2005.
Inexpensive quick meals, which may be used with rice noodles and healthier packets of seasonings.

5 a Day: Savor the Flavor of Fruits and Vegetables. Pivonka, Elizabeth, and Berry, Barbara. Rodale Books, 2003.

Short-Cut Vegetarian. Sass, Lorna. Harper Collins Publishers, 1997.
Many rave reviews on a popular bookstore website, but you may need to use a food processor to match her short-cut timing.

How Sweet It Is…Without the Sugar. Wade, Jean C. Celestial Arts, 1999.
Jean C. Wade, who has diabetes, uses fructose-based sweetener for the recipes. The cookbook has easy-to-read charts for Equivalent Sugar Substitute Measurements for natural and artificial sweeteners and lists diabetic exchanges for every recipe.

Allergy-friendly cookbooks

Vital Abundance Cooking Series #1. Falbo, Karen. Vital Abundance, 2000.
Expert certified nutritionist supplies many recipes and tips for healthful living and food allergies. Self-published. To order call 720-272-6201 or email *karenfalbo@cs.com.*

Wheat-Free Worry-Free—The Art of Happy, Healthy, Gluten-Free Living. Korn, Danna. Hay House, 2002.
This is a great wheat-free or gluten-free lifestyle nutritional information and resource directory.

The Gluten-Free Gourmet Cooks Comfort Foods: Creating Old Favorites with New Flours. Hagman, Bette. Owl Books, 2005.
Hagman authored four gluten-free books before this one. This book offers favorites such as macaroni and cheese, chicken potpie, and lasagna.

Incredible Edible Gluten-Free Food for Kids: 150 Family-Tested Recipes.
Sanderson, Sheri L. Woodbine House, 2002.
Includes recipes, tips for eating away from home, parties, trouble-shooting baker's guide, and a resource section listing gluten-free suppliers, manufacturers, and support groups.

Books for groups hardest hit with diabetes

Spirit of the Harvest: North American Indian Cooking. Cox, Beverly, and Jacobs, Martin. Stewart, Tabori & Chang, Inc, 1991.
Large historical book with lots of color photographs and recipes.

The New Soul Food Cookbook for People with Diabetes. Demps Gaines, Fabiola, and Weaver, Roniece. American Diabetes Association, 1999.

Diabetic Cooking for Latinos (Spanish): Cocinando para Latinos con diabetes. Fuste, Olga V., MS, RD. American Diabetes Association, 2002.
The Spanish classics made healthier. Includes exchanges.

On the Web

www.wholehumanbeans.com
We can unequivocally say this is the best website on the entire World Wide Web. Okay, maybe not. But this is the website for Marie's Whole Human Beans Company and we think it's pretty great. In addition to tips for healthier living, it has links to more great resources on the Internet, a place to order Marie's other books, and a Dear Waldo section with questions and answers from health-conscious parents and a form to submit your own question. In the future, Marie plans to add even more information, including some superb recipes we couldn't fit in this book, so keep checking back.

www.mypyramid.gov
This is the website for the new USDA Food Pyramid Guide for meal planning and it's absolutely packed with great information on nutrition and exercise. You may have noticed we didn't include information on the Food Pyramid in the meal planning section of this book. That's because the new Food Pyramid is designed to be personalized to each individual and is contained almost completely on this website. This is a superb resource for every family looking to eat healthier. Check it out!

www.kidshealth.org
This site is designed specifically for kids. With a focus on fun, it's filled with games to help children learn a bit about nutrition.

www.keepkidshealthy.com/nutrition/packing_school_lunches.html.
This is a great website with a variety of tips for packing lunches safely.

Mail-order grocery websites

www.vitamincottage.com
Toll free 800-817-9415
Great store whose policy is to carry products that are safe and health-promoting, while offering free nutritional education through certified nutritionists. Products with *trans* fats are not carried. Find the affordable natural ingredients listed in these recipes, as well as other gluten-free mixes, sugar-free items, and snacks. Call the Colorado shipping department for details.

www.sunorganic.com
Toll free 888-269-9888
International mail-order catalog that provides many quality ingredients, including whole-wheat pastry flour, agave, and unfumigated/unsulphured fruits.

www.netrition.com
Toll free 888-817-2411
Many nutrition products carried, including fructose, flours, bars, mixes, sugar-free products, and books. Based on the East Coast.

Other food-related websites

www.kidnetic.com
Ways to get physically fit for kids. Info such as "Totally Weird Ways to (Fruit) and Veg Out".

www.diabetes.org
Website of the American Diabetes Association. Check out this site for prevention, treatment, etc. Click on Parents & Kids for more info.

www.RD.com
Search Diabetes Update.

www.csaceliacs.org
Great celiac site with U.S.A. directory for support groups for kids and parents.

Other searches and suggested keywords
Children's nutrition games
Living without sugar
Sugarless

Websites for products we like

www.petestofu.com
This is the website for Sunrise Soya Foods in Vancouver, BC, which offers Pete's tofu. This is great for use in salads, wraps, or as is in lunchboxes. Kid-friendly divided tray to add ginger soy sauce package. For the less computer inclined, 1-800-661-BEAN.

www.nutritionlifestyles.com/waterbottles.htm
Website for the New Wave Enviro polycarbonate water bottle. Great for parents worried about plastic leaching. You can also call 1-800-592-8371 to order.

www.laptoplunches.com
Website for safe plastic modular lunchbox storage containers. The site also offers lunch ideas and news articles on healthy eating.

Food Products We Like

Keep in mind that these are products we *like*. We do not endorse any of the following food items.

Sprinkles with natural food coloring: *Sprinkelz*™, distributed by Edward & Sons Trading Co.

Ramen Noodle substitution: *Thai Kitchen's* Rice Noodles (the most popular flavor around our houses is Ginger)

Meat and Non-Meat Jerky (without nitrates): *Sheltons, Hat Creek, Vegi-Deli*

Fruits: *Good Health, Stretch Island* (fruit leather)

Healthy Snack Bars: *Govinda's Joyva, Health Valley, Pria, Nature's Choice, Clif Bars, LäraBars*

Healthy Crackers & Chips: *Edward & Sons, Hain, Lite N Krispy* (rice), *Good Health, Blue Diamond* (we like hazelnut), *Newman's Own, Little Bear*

Healthy Gluten-Free Desserts: *Westsoy, Hain, Kozy Shack, Stonyfield* (yogurt), *Jennie's* (macaroons), *Montana Moon* (cookies), *Barbara's* (animal crackers), *Glenny's* (brown rice treats), *Barbara's Fig Bars* (low sugar)

The Gluten-Free Trio

Pamela's Products   **Mrs. Leeper's**   **Edward & Sons**

This book was partially funded by an educational grant from the Gluten-Free Trio.

Index

Subject Index

A

Added sugars, 19
Agave nectar, 20
Allergy-friendly cookbooks, 135–136
All-purpose flour, 18
American diet, sugar intake, 20
Architecture, of the lunchbox, 39–40

B

Baking precision, 42
Beef, interview chart, 14
Beta carotene, 35
Bleached flour, 18
Books
  cookbooks, 37, 134–136
  for diabetics, 136
  for older children, 134
  for parents, 134
  for picky eaters, 37
  for young children, 133–134
Bread flour, 18
Breakfast, 45–47

C

Caffeine, 24
Cake flour, 18
Carbohydrates, 18–21
  fiber, 20–21, 33
  starch, 18–19
  sugar, 19–20
Charts
  food preferences, 11–16
  lunchbox-packing blueprint, 53
  menu rotation, 49–52
Chicken, interview chart, 14
Children
  books for, 133–134
  food preferences, 7–16

food preparation
   involvement, 33, 36–37
   kitchens, child-friendly, 41–43
   nutrition education for, 35–36
   picky eaters, 36–38

Cholesterol levels, 21

Cinnamon, 23

Cold food, keeping cold, 39–40

Color, added to lunches, 35

Containers, 40, 43

Cookbooks, 37, 134–136

Countertops, organization of, 43

Creativity with food, 38

D

Dairy products, interview chart, 13

Desserts, lunchbox-packing
   blueprint, 53

Diabetic diets
   beta carotene and, 35
   cookbooks, 136
   food trading and, 33

Dislikes, food. *See* Interview,
   food preferences

Divided food containers, 40

E

Education, nutrition, 35–36

Eggs, interview chart, 14

Endosperm, 18

Enriched wheat flour, 18–19

Example setting, by parents, 38

Exercise, 27

F

Fats, 21–22

Favorite foods. *See* Interview,
   food preferences

Fiber, 20–21, 33

Fish
   interview chart, 14
   mercury in, 21

Flavor, 33, 37

Flour, 18–19

Food preferences. *See* Interview,
   food preferences

Food preparation
   child involvement in, 33, 36–37
   healthy ideas for, 28
   lunch-making area,
      organizing, 41–43
   tools for, 2–3

Fruit, 24
   encouraging consumption, 25–26
   interview chart, 11
   lunchbox-packing blueprint, 53

G

Gardening, 36–37

Gluten-free diets
   baking mix, 28
   cookbooks, 135–136
   food trading and, 33

Glycemic index, 19

Grocery websites, 137

H

HDL cholesterol levels, 21

Healthy substitutes, for unhealthy
   foods, 26

Hot food, keeping hot, 39

I

Interview, food preferences, 8–16
   charts, 11–16
   suggestions for, 9–10
   supermarket stroll, 8–9
   timing/location, 8–9

Inventiveness, with food, 38

Preconceptions, negative, 37–38
Preparation. *See* Food preparation
Presentation of food, 28, 34–35
Processed foods, 18–19
Product sources, 131–138
Protein, 22
  interview chart, 14–15
  lunchbox-packing blueprint, 53
Psychology, of the lunchbox, 31–40

Q
Quick fixes, 50

R
Recipe legend, 56
Recipes. *See* **Recipe Index**
Refined grain, 18
Refrigerator organization, 43
Resources, 131–138
Reward, unhealthy food as, 36
Rotation charts, menu, 49–52

S
Salads, interview chart, 16
Saturated fats, 21
Seeds, interview chart, 15
Shapes, food preparation and, 34
Snacks
  interview chart, 16
  lunchbox-packing blueprint, 53
Social experience and food, 32
Soda pop, 24
Sprinkles, 28, 35
Starch, 18–19
Stress-busters, morning, 47

Strong flavors, toning down, 37
Substitutions, for unhealthy food, 26
Sugar, 19–20

T
Temperature, of food, 39–40
Texture variety, 37
Tools, food preparation, 2–3
Trading food, 33
Trans fats, 21

U
Uneaten food, in lunchbox, 40
Unhealthy food
  healthy substitutes for, 26
  as reward, 36

V
Variety, food, 37
Vegetables, 24
  encouraging consumption,
    25–26, 28, 36–37
  interview chart, 12
  lunchbox-packing blueprint, 53
Visual cues, from food, 34–35
Vitamins, 22–24

W
Water, 24
Weak flavors, boosting, 37
Websites, 136–138
Weekend projects, 43
Wheat, 18
Wheat flour, 18–19, 28
Whole-grains, 18, 24
Whole-wheat pastry flour, 28

Index

Recipe Index

C

Cakes
applesauce spice, 109
chocolate pound cupcakes, 129

California (Nori) Rolls, 78

Carrot or Zucchini Muffins, 1262

Carrot soup, 84

Celery Stuffing, 97

Chicken
crunchy baked, 82
pecan-crusted, 87
stew, hominy thick, 83
tangy, with peanut butter dipping
sauce, 64
tortellini salad, 85

Chinese rolled pancakes, 67

Chocolate Chip Cookies, 114

Chocolate pound cupcakes, 129

Cinderella Pumpkin Soup, 74

Coleslaw
fruit, 99
honey peanut, 100
kidney bean, 101

Cookies
chocolate chip, 114
fortune, 125
oatmeal, 113
peanut butter sandwich, 110
shortbread jam, 123

Corn dip, 105

Corny Cornbread, 116

Crock pot recipes
bean dip, 102
steak soup, 77

Crunchy Munchy Lunchy Chicken, 82

Cupcakes, chocolate pound, 129

D

Deli Fajita, 65

Desserts. *See also* **Cakes; Cookies**
apricot-pineapple pie, 120–121
brownies, 122
brown rice pudding, 127
pumpkin pie, 120–121
pumpkin pudding, 124

Dips
bean, 102
corn, 105
eggplant, 69
peach and peanut butter, 96
peanut butter dipping sauce, 64
polenta, 104

E

Easy Chinese Rolled Pancakes, 67

Easy English Muffin Pizza, 91

Eggplant dip, 69

Eskimo Ice Cream, 93

F

Fab Brownies, 122

Fajitas, 65

Fake 'n' Bake Pecan-Crusted Chicken, 87

Fit for a King Applesauce Spice Cake, 109

Fortune cookies, 125

Frozen yogurt, 93

Fruit
applesauce spice cake, 109
apricot-pineapple pie, 120–121
banana nut bread, 112
banana split, 95

pinwheels
  Mexican, 70
  vegetable, 71
  vegetable filling, marinated, 80
Sauces
  peach and peanut butter
    dipping, 96
  peanut butter dipping sauce, 64
Seafood
  shrimp party plate, 68
Shortbread Jam Cookies, 123
Shrimp Party Plate, 68
Side dishes.
  See **Fruit; Vegetables**
Snacks. *See also* **Dips**
  banana nut bread, 112
  banana split, lunchbox, 95
  bran muffins, honey, 117
  bread, fried, 115
  brown rice pudding, 127
  carrot muffins, 126
  celery, stuffed, 97
  cornbread, 116
  English muffin pizza, 91
  frozen yogurt and fruit, 93
  fruit leather, 92
  fruit muffins, 118
  granola bars, 119
  party mix, 103
  polenta, with bell pepper
    strips, 104
  raisin bean muffins, 128
  sweet potato knots, 111
  zucchini muffins, 126
(Sort of) Ramen Nachos, 76
Soups
  butternut squash, 62
  carrot, 84
  chicken hominy thick stew, 83

pumpkin, 74
steak, 77
Spice cake, applesauce, 109
Spicy Mac 'n' Cheese with
  Broccoli, 79
Spicy Raisin Bean Muffins, 128
Steak soup, 77
Stew, chicken hominy, 83
Stuffed celery, 97
Super-Duper Muffins, 118
Sweet potato knots, 111
Sweet snacks. *See* **Cookies;
  Desserts; Snacks**

T

Tawny Scrawny Lion Carrot Soup, 84
Thumbs-up Easy Chocolate Pound
  Cupcakes, 129
Tortellini salads
  chicken, 85
  lentil, 88
  vegetable, 86
Tortillas
  Chinese rolled pancakes, 67
  fajitas, deli, 65
  pinwheels
    Mexican, 70
    vegetable, 71
Turkey Lurkey Jerky, 75

V

Vegetables
  bell pepper, with polenta dip, 104
  broccoli
    macaroni and cheese, 79
    -raisin salad, 98

Other Titles Available from Small Steps Press

Disease Prevention Cookbook
By Clara Schneider, MS, RD, RN, LD, CDE
This innovative cookbook is filled with delicious recipes and tools designed to help you prevent some of the most prevalent diseases in our society, including diabetes, heart disease, stroke, and cancer.
Order #4651-01
$14.95 US

Small Steps, Big Rewards: Walking Your Way to Better Health
By Small Steps Press
A pedometer and book combo, this kit is the perfect start for those looking to enjoy better health.
Order #5012-01
$19.95 US

200 Healthy Recipes in 30 Minutes—Or Less!
By Robyn Webb
Renowned cookbook author Robyn Webb has scoured her bestsellers and compiled the tastiest, quickest, and easiest recipes into one fabulous book.
Order #4654-01
$16.95 US

Dr. Gavin's Health Guide for African Americans
By James Gavin, PhD, MD, with Sherrye Landrum
This all-in-one guide focuses on the health issues that most affect African Americans.
Order #4870-01
$14.95 US

To order these and other great Small Steps Press titles, call 1-800-232-6733
or visit http://store.diabetes.org. Small Steps Press titles are
also available in bookstores nationwide.

SMALL STEPS PRESS